Marketing Health/Fitness Services

Marketing Health/Fitness Services

Richard F. Gerson, PhD
Gerson, Goodson, Inc.
Safety Harbor, Florida

Human Kinetics Books
Champaign, Illinois

Library of Congress Cataloging-in-Publication Data
Gerson, Richard F.
    Marketing health/fitness services.

    Bibliography: p.
    Includes index.
    1. Physical fitness centers—Management.
2. Physical fitness—Marketing. 3. Medical care—
Marketing. I. Title.
GV428.5.G47   1989   613.7'068   88-13078
ISBN 0-87322-931-2

Developmental Editor: Lisa Busjahn
Production Director: Ernie Noa
Copy Editor: Bruce Owens
Proofreader: Phaedra Hise
Assistant Editor: Holly Gilly
Typesetter: Cindy Pritchard
Text Design: Keith Blomberg
Cover Designer: Hunter Graphics
Text Layout: Jayne Clampitt
Printed By: Braun Brumfield

ISBN: 0-87322-931-2

Printed in the United States of America

10 9 8 7 6 5 4 3 2 1

Human Kinetics Books
A Division of Human Kinetics Publishers, Inc.
Box 5076, Champaign, IL 61820
1-800-DIAL-HKP
1-800-334-3665 (in Illinois)

This book is dedicated in loving memory to my grandfather, Joe Schuster, whose inspiration for achievement will always be with me and whose marketing advice was simply ''Keep on punching, kid!'' It works.

Contents _____

Preface _____

In presenting marketing seminars to health and fitness professionals, I have found that many have devoted so much time to learning about their areas of specialization they haven't taken time to learn the language and organizational structure of business and marketing. This information is necessary to planning and operating any successful business. If clearly presented, business and marketing procedures can be easily acquired and implemented.

The ideas in this book are drawn from my 10 years of experience owning and directing a financially successful health/fitness consulting business that offers services in stress management, weight control, risk reduction, time management, and other areas. I have also applied my experience in directing hospital, health club, and community health programs in marketing decision-making processes.

I feel the best way to teach you what I have learned is to take you step by step through writing a comprehensive business and marketing plan. Your gathering the information needed to complete these plans ensures that your marketing decisions will be based on complete, up-to-date information. By writing out your plans you create core documents that you can show to prospective clients, investors, and new employees.

As you read the book, you will notice that certain words are italicized, which means that they are defined in the glossary at the back of the book. Please refer to the glossary as you read, for you need to understand the terminology to effectively write and implement your business and marketing plans.

Chapter 1 outlines the steps you need to take before writing a business plan, including doing, or hiring someone to do, initial marketing research. Both the nature of this research and examples of its application are described. Seven questions are listed that you should ask yourself to help specify your company's goals, objectives, and directions.

In chapter 2 you will learn how the components of the business plan fit together to create a comprehensive description of the methods you will use to attain your goals and objectives. This chapter provides in-depth explanations of the business plan components that relate to the company, to its position in the immediate competitive market, and to its relation to the health and fitness industry as a whole. These first four components are the executive summary, the company analysis, the industry analysis, and the market analysis.

Chapter 3 details the strategic, management, and financial analyses. These components are keys to decisions you will face regarding your current and projected management structure. A sample business plan illustrates how all the business plan components work together to shape a clear and specific management plan.

Your business plan provides information that is crucial to developing a successful marketing plan. Chapter 4 describes the process of writing the marketing plan and how to incorporate pertinent information already gathered for the business plan. For example, you will see how your market analysis depends on information included in your business plan's competitive analysis.

Chapter 5 discusses how to determine your promotional goals, methods, and expenditures and explains how your marketing budget and promotional strategies and tactics influence each other. For instance, if you are marketing a new product with a limited budget, you will make different decisions than if you are marketing an established product with a large promotional budget. Developing promotional plans is imperative to completing a marketing plan. Chapter 5 outlines two sample marketing plans—one for a company that sells a product and another for a company that offers a service in the form of a fitness facility. The similarities and differences of these plans will help clarify how each component of a marketing plan must be tailored to the individual company, product, and market.

Chapter 6 teaches you how to develop a personal approach to sales. Although the personal sales approach is part of the promotional mix, your own sales style will influence many promotional decisions to such a degree that it is important to expand on this component of the mix. Chapter 6 explains the six steps to making a sale: prospecting, making the approach, presenting the product, handling objections, closing the sale, and following up on customer satisfaction. An example of the personal approach to selling a service shows you how these steps relate to sales challenges you may face.

I am confident you will find the information and examples collected here valuable to your future in the business world. Now, let's get down to business!

Acknowledgments

It is difficult to write a book of this type without a great deal of help from many people. I thank those who had a tremendous influence on the outcome of this book. If I have forgotten anyone, it is simply my error, but my gratitude is not lessened because I may have omitted their names. They know who they are and how much I appreciate their efforts and involvement.

I want to begin by thanking the editorial staff at Human Kinetics Publishers, especially Lisa Busjahn and Sue Wilmoth, who spent many hours guiding me in the right direction for this book. I also want to thank Dr. Neil Sol for his helpful comments on a draft of the book and Scott McWilliams, president of Scott McWilliams Marketing Services in Tampa, Florida, for his help with the information on market research that appears in this book.

The people and organizations with whom I have consulted over the years have also played a role in this book's development as it was their projects to which I applied these basic marketing principles and found that they work in the health and fitness industry. My gratitude is also extended to SPRI Products for allowing me to include its marketing plan as an example in this book.

Finally, this book could never have been written without the total support and love of my family. My wife, Robbie, and my son, Michael, endured long hours and months of my writing and editing. They gave up many family activities so that I could finish the book. Now that it is complete, I want them to know that they have my ultimate gratitude and undying love. Thank you so much.

Chapter 1

Preparing to Write Your Business Plan _____

The first thing to do before launching any new business venture or updating an existing one is to develop a *business plan**. A business plan describes why the business or program should be developed and exactly what must be done to ensure its successful implementation. It is necessary because it explains why the programs are to be developed, what the *goals* are, how they will be achieved, and how long it will take to achieve them. The plan is also a guide that helps to minimize the risks and maximize the opportunities for and potentials of marketing programs, products, or services. The entire business plan is an outgrowth of the *market research* process, the results of which determine whether you should proceed with a venture or the development of a program.

The Market Research Process

Market research involves investigating the qualitative and quantitative probabilities of success for a new program, service, product, or business. You do this by trying to identify potential *customers—*your *market—*and then finding out what their needs, likes, and dislikes are. Next, through statistical analyses of their responses, you determine which program, product, or service they are most likely to buy to satisfy those needs.

Market research is defined as the systematic process of gathering, analyzing, interpreting, and utilizing relevant information for the purpose of making accurate *marketing* decisions (Murphy & Enis, 1985). The

---

*Italicized words appear in the glossary at the back of the book.

1

objectives of this process include understanding consumer behavior and perceptions; providing specific, verifiable, hard data about a market place (Reibstein, 1985); developing an ongoing marketing information system; identifying potential customers for health and fitness services; determining which factors will reduce the risk of offering these services; and measuring the effectiveness with which previous services have been provided. Market research is basically the measurement component of marketing.

A Scientific Method

The market research process is similar to the scientific method in that the five steps described must be followed:

1. Identification and definition of a problem
2. The situational analysis, which includes the research design
3. The collection of data
4. The analysis and interpretation of the data
5. The solution to the problem and recommendations for further action (cf. Murphy & Enis, 1985)

But Reibstein (1985) suggests that before a company engages in a market research program, three criteria are met: (a) There is uncertainty about a particular marketing decision. (b) The company is prepared to change its direction or focus in response to the research results. (c) The cost of the research will not exceed the research's potential value to the business. If these criteria are not met, then it may not be necessary to do a market research study.

Most health and fitness professionals are familiar with market research studies that are completed prior to opening a facility or offering a service. These feasibility studies are designed to determine the financial viability of a project. You should remember that market research is an ongoing process that must be performed both when you are offering the service and after it is adopted by the customer. For example, suppose you conduct a needs assessment (feasibility study) of corporations in your area related to their desire to adopt health and fitness programs. You find out that 75% of the companies questioned are interested in starting some type of program. After you provide the program, you distribute evaluation questionnaires which will help you determine your program's effectiveness and what your customers may want or need in the future.

Data Collection

Market research is only as valuable as the data that are collected and the techniques used to gather those data. Market researchers use *secondary data* and *primary data* to help in making decisions. You collect your secondary data first because these are data that are most easily accessible and least expensively collected.

Secondary Data. Secondary data are those that have been collected usually for purposes not related to your project (Assael, 1985). Internal sources of secondary data include company files, financial reports, marketing information systems, and employees. External sources include government publications, competitors' publications, trade associations and publications, libraries, research organizations, universities, censuses, Dun and Bradstreet reports, sales and marketing management surveys, and informed people.

There are both advantages and disadvantages of using secondary data in your market research. The advantages are that they save time and money and prevent a duplication of effort. The disadvantages are that the data may not apply to the situation under study, the data may be outdated, or the available data may be uninterpretable (Reibstein, 1985). Also, secondary data must be carefully evaluated for their relevancy, credibility, and accuracy before being used (Murphy & Enis, 1985). As long as the advantages outweigh the disadvantages, you should proceed with primary data collection.

Primary Data. Primary data are those you collect yourself to analyze your specific situation. These data can be either qualitative (subjective) or quantitative (measurable). Qualitative information is gathered, for example, through focus groups to determine *consumer* attitudes and preferences toward your health and fitness services, through interviews, and through published statements related to your inquiries. Quantitative data are much more reliable because statistical analyses can be performed on them. Sources of quantitative data include surveys either in person, on the telephone (*telemarketing*), or through the mail (*direct mail*); observing behavior, using criterion reference points to score consumer actions; and case studies. The results of the analysis on these hard data, combined with the qualitative primary and available secondary data, will help you make more accurate marketing decisions.

Recording and Evaluating Data

As mentioned previously, marketing research is an ongoing process that should be performed before you develop the business and marketing plans, during the implementation of these plans, and afterward as you evaluate the effectiveness of your efforts. Many companies neglect to perform research because they feel it is too expensive. Although it is true that the costs of marketing research are time, money, and the risk in relation to outcome, these costs are usually less than those of not doing market research and then proceeding with a new venture with no support information.

The results of the market research process are usually included in the business and marketing plans. You should prepare a separate market research report for each project undertaken. Murphy and Enis (1985) suggest that the report include

- a title page;
- a table of contents;
- an executive summary;
- an introduction;
- a body (including methodology);
- results and study limitations;
- conclusions and recommendations;
- an appendix with data collection forms, statistics, and tables not included in the body of the report; and
- a bibliography or reference list.

A separate report will allow others easy access to your research and results, and it can also serve as a secondary data source for a different project.

A final suggestion must be made regarding market research. It is usually better for a health and fitness company to use the services of a professional market research firm rather than to try to perform the study itself. The marketing research firm has the data collection and statistical analysis capabilities as this is usually its sole line of business. Have one of these firms handle the market research projects that are larger in scope than your company is capable of handling. The added expense will be worth it as the results will help you make or save money in the long run. Once your market research has been accomplished, you can begin formulating your business plan. The business plan contains seven major components, which will be described in detail in chapter 2. First, we will take a brief look at the basic functions of the business plan.

Functions of the Business Plan

Traditionally, a business plan serves four important functions:

- It describes the company's goals, objectives, implementation target dates, *strategies, tactics,* and potential for success in given market.
- It enables potential clients, customers, corporate officers, and bankers or creditors to assess the talents of the program director as a business manager.
- It serves as a communication tool that familiarizes clients and employees with the company's goals and method of operation.

- It is an organized approach to developing your own management skills as you define company or program assets and liabilities, describe competitive and market conditions, identify facility and financial needs, predict problems and devise appropriate solutions, and identify strategies and tactics that will lead to success.

Meeting the challenge of writing a comprehensive plan that fulfills each of these functions begins when you ask yourself basic questions about the nature of your business, product or service, market, competition, and proposed methods of distribution.

Seven Preliminary Questions

There are seven questions that must be addressed when developing the business plan to ensure that the basic functions of the plan are effectively carried out. The responses to these questions can be used to focus the plan toward desired goals and objectives.

What Is the Nature of the Business?

Anyone trying to develop a health and fitness program—especially those in a for-profit venture—is selling a service first and a product or program second. You must identify the type of service that is being offered. Some examples are facility design, program development, personnel recruitment, staff development and training, class instruction, operations management, or simply exercise classes.

Where Is My Market Located?

Decide where (geographically), how (physically), and to whom (demograpically) services and programs will be offered. Will the market concentration be within a 5- or 10-mile radius of your facility, in an urban or a rural setting, or in a corporation? Will these services and programs be offered locally or on a county, state, regional, or national level?

When Are Services and Programs Distributed?

You should not haphazardly enter the business of providing services as poor or untimely provisions of services will almost always lead to failure. For example, assume that you have informed your clients or employees that a 4-week stress management program is available when in reality you only have a 2-hour lecture prepared. Now, to make matters worse, the client wants the program delivered immediately. Obviously, you cannot turn a 2-hour lecture into a quality 4-week program overnight.

Who Are the Competitors and What Are They Doing?

Know who your *competitors* are, what services they provide, and what their strengths and weaknesses are. For example, if you are directing a hospital-based health and fitness program and plan to offer health promotion classes to selected segments of the community, you must know what the other hospitals in the area are offering in comparison to what you want to offer. You should know what programs they offer, when they offer them, and how much the programs cost. This information will help you plan your business and marketing strategies more intelligently.

Who Are the Customers?

Define and describe the customer market. Will it be company employees? Individuals in the community? Corporations, hospitals, and community organizations? Be specific in identifying customer characteristics as these will determine your marketing approach, the services that will be purchased or used, and how the services will be provided.

How Will the Services and Programs Be Distributed?

When services are provided in community settings by for-profit organizations, or even by nonprofit companies such as YMCAs and some hospitals, the distribution method is predetermined. But services that are distributed within a corporate fitness program, for example, are usually based on time and the availability of people and facilities. You must schedule the delivery of the service (e.g., by personal contact, lecture, programmed text, or electronic media) well in advance. Remember that clients will usually need to arrange their schedules to use the service.

What Are the Financial Requirements of the Business?

Financial planning must include *development costs, operational expenses,* predicted revenue generation, *cash flow* estimates, and profitability measures. Proper financial planning provides an accurate estimate of the funds needed to start the business or offer the program even in times of minimal cash flow.

The answers to these questions serve as an outline for developing a more comprehensive business plan. Turn now to chapter 2, which discusses writing the formal plan.

The First Four Business Plan Components _____

The business plan is one of the two most important documents needed to operate a successful health and fitness business. It is the foundation for much of the marketing plan, which is the second key document. Because of its importance two chapters are devoted to explaining the sections of the business plan. In chapter 2 I present the sections that relate to the company, its relation to the health and fitness industry as a whole, and its position in the immediate competitive market. These sections of the business plan are the *executive summary*, the *company analysis*, the *industry analysis*, and the *market analysis*.

The information you gather to complete each section of the business plan influences decisions you will make about the primary goals of your business. Thus, it is important to keep each section in mind as you work on the next one and in light of your total plan. The following list of the major components to the business plan will help you understand how each section contributes to the whole and will guide you in writing your own plan.

Major Components of a Business Plan

I. Executive Summary

   A. General description of the business plan

   B. Introduction to the company

   C. Brief description of the marketing program

   D. Business and financial goals and requirements

II. Company Analysis

   A. SWOT analysis

   B. Company history

   C. Product, program, and service offerings

   D. Prospective markets and clients

   E. Technology and resources

   F. Major competitors and competitive position

   G. Success factors

   H. Cost comparisons

III. Industry Analysis

   A. Definition of the industry

   B. Growth rate

   C. Key growth factors

   D. Financial operating characteristics

   E. Industry product life cycle

IV. Market Analysis

   A. Market scope

   B. Market segmentation

   C. Market barriers

   D. Market demand and market share

   E. Market sales

   F. Sales tactics and distribution channels

   G. Price structures and policies

   H. Advertising and promotion

V. Strategic Analysis

   A. Goals and objectives

   B. Key performance indicators

C. Project completion schedule

D. Operating assumptions

VI. Management Analysis

A. Identification of management personnel

B. Personnel pro forma

C. Organizational structure

D. Management philosophy

VII. Financial Analysis

A. Budgets

B. Financial schedules and statements

Let us begin by examining the first component of a business plan, the executive summary, and the elements that contribute to its completion.

The Executive Summary

An executive summary should concisely describe the entire business plan. You can use the executive summary with investors, prospective clients, new employees, and others to give a clear encapsulation of your goals and your plans for reaching them. This summary is usually between two and four pages long.

An executive summary typically begins with a *mission statement*—one to three sentences describing your company's goals and objectives. For example, the mission statement for a health and fitness provider might be

> The company intends to be a health and fitness service provider that attains a 10% *market share* through personal sales of stress management and relaxation programs and thorough customer-satisfaction follow-up.

This statement tells the reader exactly what the company wants to do and how. Of course, your mission statement needs to be tailored to your business.

The rest of the executive summary follows the mission statement. The summary is, in effect, a mini-business plan; it should include the following elements:

- A definition of the business
- A statement of organizational philosophy and commitment

- The *differentiation* of the services from those of competitors
- A description of the working environment
- A statement of provisions for effective response to change, including marketing and financial alternatives
- Financial planning statements
- The geographic service area
- The provision of services
- The level, range, and scope of services
- Company strengths and competencies
- Company weaknesses and limitations
- Outside agency and institutional relationships/networks
- Organizational management
- Human resource management
- Expansion and growth opportunities

A clear, concise yet comprehensive summary will make a positive impact while capturing the reader's attention and setting the tone for all the material that follows.

The Company Analysis

The next section of the business plan is the company analysis, also called the internal environment analysis or the corporate environment analysis. The purpose of the company analysis is to provide a critical, objective look at the company either as it presently is or as it will be in the future as the materials in this section serve as a basis for other items in the plan.

The SWOT Analysis

The simplest form of a company analysis is called a *SWOT analysis*, which stands for *Strengths, Weaknesses, Opportunities,* and *Threats.* The SWOT analysis identifies the firm's Strengths, such as financial, product delivery, or personnel; its Weaknesses, such as a lack of capital, or a lack of current clients; the Opportunities that are available for successful performance, such as lower prices, new product development, or a competitor going out of business; and the Threats, such as competitors having lower-priced programs and services, other new companies being formed, or unrealistic performance goals set by management. These are only some of the possible components of a SWOT analysis. Others can be included. The sample form provided here can be used to develop a SWOT analysis.

SWOT Analysis

Strengths	Weaknesses
Opportunities	Threats

The SWOT analysis can be included as additional support material if you decide to write a comprehensive company analysis. Writing an in-depth analysis will provide you with more information from which to make intelligent business and marketing decisions.

The Comprehensive Analysis

A comprehensive analysis provides a complete profile of your company and close competitors. It requires that you gather the following information.

Historical Data. These explain how and why your company was formed, how well it has performed in the past, and the philosophical ideas that led to its formation.

Products and Services. These are the marketable, or salable, services that will be provided for clients. Every service should be described in detail so that a marketing and sales strategy can be developed for each.

Markets. This section briefly describes the company's potential clients, the unique characteristics they may possess, and why you think they will buy your services.

Technology Position. How sophisticated the programs and services will be must be decided on and described. Will the programs be computerized, or will programmed text be used? Will *follow-up* service be in person or by telephone? These are some of the questions that must be answered when defining your technology position.

Operational Resources. These are all the resources—including internal personnel, external suppliers and vendors, and available finances—that can be used to provide health and fitness services to clients. The scope and availability of a program is often limited not by the resourcefulness of the director and the staff but by external influences such as facilities and finances that affect how a program is presented.

Competitors. This section describes the competitors or those providing similar programs and services. A *competitor analysis* can be done through financial, stock, and sales reports as well as through available personnel and archival data. Each competitor's relative position in the market must be determined.

Company Strengths and Weaknesses. These must be identified in as critical a manner as possible. It is always helpful to use the SWOT analysis as a starting point. However, taking a critical look at your company or programs is not always easy to do, especially for a new director. All company analyses should be done as if done by a competitor. After all, when you analyze a competitor, you are looking for weaknesses that can be exploited to your benefit. Analyzing your company or programs as if you were the chief competitor will give you a more objective and useful report.

Success Factors. Identify factors such as finances, products, programs, services, or staff performance, which are the keys to your company's success. It is helpful to determine levels of success related to both program and company goals. For example, will an exercise program sold to a company of 100 employees be considered a success if only 20 people participate in the program? Or must a greater number of people in the company participate to generate a certain amount of revenue for you to consider the program a success? Similarly, will an acceptable level of participation in a smoking-cessation program be 10% of all smokers in a company, or must 75% to 100% of the smokers participate before the implementation of the program is considered successful?

To identify levels of success, determine which levels are needed for outstanding success (75% to 100% participation rate), respectable success (25% to 74%), and acceptable success (10% to 24%). It is helpful to use these levels as you determine the financial requirements that will make your company or program a success. Must you break even during the first year, or will you allow 3 to 5 years for profitability? Answers to these questions will also help set goals and improve the financial analysis processes that are described later in the business plan.

Cost Comparisons. Cost comparison means identifying the *prices* of products, programs, and services being offered by competitors. Compare these prices with those being planned for similar offerings by your company.

Competitive Position. *Competitive position* is based on the competitors' market share and the methods your company will use to obtain its own level of market share. You must describe where your company currently fits in the market. Then you must describe what will be done to maintain or improve this position. Remember that if you are directing a corporate health and fitness program, your client base is the employees of the company. You should analyze competitors for this client base just as you would if your client base were in the community.

Often a strong competitive position in a small *market niche* is more desirable than is a large market share. This strong position can be achieved by offering lower-priced and higher quality services, and better follow-up than your competition offers. Only the company's management can determine where and how to position the company. The same principles hold true for a company health promotion program.

Again, the company analysis should be as complete as possible to provide guidance throughout the operation of the business. The company analysis is followed by the industry analysis. A program director who is writing a business plan can keep the industry analysis section brief as fluctuations in the industry as a whole will probably not affect program offerings within a corporation. On the other hand, the director of a new or expanding health and fitness service business must carefully scrutinize the entire industry to determine how to make a positive impact.

The Industry Analysis

The purpose of the industry analysis is to create a comprehensive picture of the health and fitness industry. The focus is on the industry in general, not on one specific competitor, although it is sometimes difficult not to analyze your chief competitor too. The industry analysis will help determine fluctuations in the market, whether the industry is strong or weak, when a move should be made to carve a new or larger niche in the industry, and the health and fitness industry's operating characteristics.

There are four major areas that must be covered by the industry analysis: service definition, growth rate/key growth factors, financial operating characteristics, and industry/product life cycle. Each must be researched thoroughly to provide information for the rest of the business plan and for the entire marketing plan.

Service Definition

You must define accurately the scope of the health and fitness service industry that your company or programs will most significantly affect. If you are developing health promotion programs, are you going to provide clients with a range of programs, or will you focus on one or two such as stress management and weight control? Narrow your definition of the industry, but remember that the definition should refer to the relative size of the industry, the characteristics of its consumers, other providers in your portion of the industry, and your personal views of the industry. This last item may be the most important to include because you will most likely run your programs in the way you see as most effective.

Growth Rate/Key Growth Factors

You must determine the growth rate of your area of the health and fitness industry and identify the key factors that influence that growth. The growth rate is determined by identifying the number of providers for a given number of consumers as well as by analyzing information from trade journals or shows, stock reports, financial reports, and surveys of industry leaders. Your original market research will also provide you with information about how well your programs fit into the chosen market. Industry growth factors are readily identifiable and include factors such as more people becoming involved in physical activity, more companies developing employee wellness programs, and more people living longer who need health promotion information to maintain the quality of their lives.

Financial Operating Characteristics

You must specify the methods by which transactions occur in the industry as a whole. Most providers prefer to be paid in cash for programs or services at the time they are provided. However, many consumers prefer to buy on credit. Evaluate how the industry operates financially, and how your company fits into this scheme. Also, determine whether you will provide discounts for early payments and penalties for late payments. How the industry handles these factors must be clearly identified so that you can develop pricing structures and policies in relation to it.

Industry/Product Life Cycle

Every health and fitness product, program, or service goes through a series of stages from the time it is introduced until the time it is removed from the market. The *industry/product life cycle* depicts the rate of sales growth, plateau, and eventual decline in the life of a program, product, service, or company. There are four stages to the industry/product life cycle: introduction, growth, maturity, and decline (see Figure 2.1).

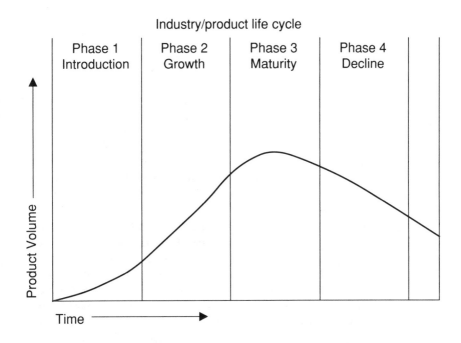

Figure 2.1. The four stages of the industry/product life cycle: introduction, growth, maturity, and decline.

Each stage has a unique set of marketing strategies associated with it (Rink & Swan, 1987). Current evidence indicates that the health and fitness industry is still in the initial phases of the growth stage, which means that companies should try to expand by gaining a greater market niche or share. This assumption is supported by the fact that more people are entering the market place, and more corporations are establishing employee health and fitness programs. The industry should remain strong for many years to come.

Next, you must identify the factors that will keep the industry in its current stage or move it to the next one. Some of these include the demand for the product, program, or service; the availability of competing or substitute products; the pricing of the services; and the promotional efforts of the providers. If the industry becomes oversaturated with any of these products, programs, or services or if the supply of health and fitness services begins to exceed the demand, then the industry will move into the maturation phase and will require a new set of survival strategies. The industry analysis identifies the current status of the health and fitness industry and the possible future directions in which it can move. This analysis, when combined with the company analysis, leads the way to a more thorough understanding of the market place, and so will assist you as you write your market analysis.

The Market Analysis

The market analysis determines the critical path your company will follow to identify and secure clients, sell and distribute its programs and services, advertise and promote itself, allocate personnel and other resources to specific marketing tasks, and forecast sales goals. The market analysis will also help the company deterimine the ease with which it can enter or exit a particular market (Bennett, 1988; Crego, Deaton, & Schiffrin, 1986; Kotler, 1988) and what type of market share it can expect to achieve from its efforts.

The market analysis should begin with a statement of purpose that is based on the results of your market research. Remember that you did market research to find a need for starting your business or implementing your program. The results of the research need to be mentioned first to set the tone for the rest of the plan. Then the market analysis must be written comprehensively enough to include all the information mentioned above and concisely enough so that it is not mistaken for the more formal *marketing plan*. The marketing plan uses the market analysis as a foundation for its development. But remember that the market analysis only looks at the markets in which the company plans to do business. It is not a detailed specification of the activities and techniques that the company will engage in to achieve its goals.

Market Scope and Segmentation

Market scope refers to the areas within which a company offers its services. These can be departments within a company, or they can be geographical areas such as local, state, regional, or national markets. Most new businesses in the health and fitness industry should consider beginning on a local or state level, mainly because it often requires too much capital to start on a regional or national level. Starting small makes it easier both to maintain more control of all aspects of the business or program and to achieve some early success.

Market segmentation is perhaps one of the most important features of the market analysis. Segmentation refers to methods by which groups of prospective clients or, in the case of a corporate health and fitness program, employees are distinguished from other customers. The distinctions are made according to a set of common characteristics possessed by one group but not by another. Some of the characteristics used to segment a market follow.

Geography.   This refers to a region, a particular locale, a county or city, population density, corporate density, and climate. It is usually classified as an area where people live and work.

Demographics.   These are the most common characteristics that are used to segment a market. *Demographics* include age, sex, marital status, family size, personal and household income, people per household, education, occupation, culture, religion, nationality, job requirements, leisure activities, and socioeconomic status. Although there are other demographic factors, these are the primary ones.

Psychographics.   These factors include lifestyle, personality, purchasing behaviors, product/service usage rate, degree of loyalty to a product brand or even an employer, benefits sought from the items purchased or from the job, and job change rate. Psychographics is also called sociographics, but this distinction is usually arbitrary.

These factors help to define a market segment. The same marketing approach will not be effective for each market segment. Each segment may require its own marketing approach, and each approach may require a differentiation of services. If you carefully plan and analyze market segmentation, then identifying and implementing the appropriate marketing approaches will be clearer to you as you develop your marketing plan. Taking the time to plan at this point will ensure most of the programs and services you are offering will reach their intended markets. An additional way to secure the connection between services, programs, and market is to answer the following questions:

- Are there enough people or companies in the proposed market segment to make entry and penetration worthwhile?
- Do the people or companies in this market segment recognize their need for our programs and services? Or, can they be educated to recognize their needs and our ability to satisfy those needs?
- Do the potential clients have the ability to pay for the programs and services?
- Can the potential clients be reached through our marketing and advertising approaches?

Each of these questions must be answered "yes" if you are to penetrate a chosen market successfully. Barriers to market penetration must be realistically anticipated before any attempt is made to enter a particular market.

Market Barriers

Several barriers to both market entry and market exit must be identified so that you can make realistic time and budget projections regarding each. The major *market barriers* will be described and explained in the following sections.

Market Entry Barriers. Market entry barriers include the minimum volume or number of resources your company or program must use to run a cost-effective business, the differentiation of programs and services, competitors in each market segment, and consumer perceptions of the program or service as a unique one. Financial requirements can also serve as barriers to market entry. These include expenditures for facilities, equipment, furniture, program development, and advertising as well as for production and proposed operating costs. Other barriers you must consider include the costs incurred by clients when they switch from one provider to another, the ability of your company to access suppliers or vendors, the laws that govern licensing and operating the business or selling the programs, and the cost disadvantages of being a new entrant in the market (your costs will probably be higher than those of a company that has been in the market for a longer period of time).

Market Exit Barriers. Barriers to market entry are counterbalanced by barriers to market exit. Market exit occurs when a program or service is no longer profitable due possibly to high delivery costs or oversaturation of the market with competitors. This usually happens in the maturation or in the decline phase of the industry life cycle, when the company decides to get out of the business.

Two other major barriers to market exit are a strong desire by management to continue offering a service despite a decline in customers, revenue, or profits and the relationship of the product or service to other components of the business. If the service can be provided as a *loss leader*, to sell other higher-priced services to clients, then you may find it difficult to exit the market, even when clients continue to purchase only your lower-priced program. The temptation is to continue to offer the program, hoping that someone will buy a higher-priced service with it. For example, your company may offer a low-priced stress management program to a major company in hopes that the company will then buy more expensive physical examinations. This is a legitimate sales technique, but you must ask whether your company is using it at a time the program should be exiting the market.

Market Demand

Recently, there have been many changes in the demand for health and fitness services. Businesses are establishing programs for their employees; there has been an increase in the number of fitness centers and businesses that provide health and fitness programs; there have been changes in the relative sizes of the *target markets* (i.e., all age groups are becoming involved in health and fitness) and in the geographic distribution of the markets as people become mobile and want to continue their fitness programs wherever they work, live, or travel; new market segments have emerged (e.g., children, the elderly, and the physically challenged); and clients have begun to request new and more advanced services such as computerized testing equipment and computer-aided instruction. You must identify the *market demand* characteristics that are pertinent to your program, service offerings, or company.

Market Share

The demand for a service will also influence predicting the market share that can be achieved. Market share refers to the percentage of all potential clients who use one company's services. It is like owning a portion of the health and fitness industry. Every company must determine its present and desired market share, which is usually determined by one of the four following methods:

- As a percentage of all service users for a defined geographic area (How many people who use health and fitness services are using *your* services?)

- As a percentage of service users from a specifically defined segment of a target market (e.g., 50% of the overweight employees in your company having registered for a weight-control program)
- As a percentage of a competitor's defined market segment or geographical area for a selected service or program activity (i.e., you have successfully entered a competitor's service area and attracted a certain percentage of participants to your program. Buzzell and Gale [1987] refer to this as relative market share.)
- As a percentage of all service users on a national basis (basically the same as the previous method, but on a much wider scale)

The best method for a company to use must be decided on by its management. Market share, along with profits, is often used as the measure of a company's success. But two companies can offer the same service and use different definitions of market share, yet one will be considered successful and the other unsuccessful. You must always "compare apples with apples" when you use market share to measure your company against a competitor.

Market Sales

Market sales and revenue are the estimated sales—either in the number of programs or services sold or in dollar amounts—that a company provides to a specific target market within a given time frame. Estimates of market sales are based on the number of clients a company services or expects to service, the client's acceptance of the programs or services, the renewal or repurchase rates of those services, and competitors' sales. Sales and revenue should be forecast monthly, annually, and multiannually. Figure 2.2 shows a sample monthly sales forecast.

You can more accurately predict revenue figures if you can identify qualified prospects in addition to your current clients. You can then categorize them as major or minor customers based on demographics, purchasing power, their program needs, and the percentage of sales they represent. This will help you determine how much time to spend trying to sell your services to each client, the types of sales tactics to use to approach the clients (or employees if you direct a corporate health and fitness program), and the closing techniques to use to help make the sale.

Tactics and Distribution Channels

You must describe the sales methods you will use to get the consumer to purchase your programs and services. These include personal selling, direct mail, telephone sales (telemarketing), company representatives, and

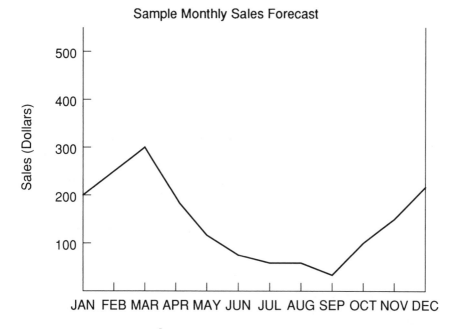

Figure 2.2. Sample 12-month monthly sales forecast.

distributors. It will also help to compare your sales program to those of your competitors.

Most producers of goods and services use middlemen as *distribution channels* for their products. Middlemen buy consumer goods at wholesale prices and then sell them to the final purchaser at retail prices. The middlemen in the fitness equipment industry are the retail outlets that sell home fitness equipment; they buy the equipment directly from the manufacturer and sell it to someone else. Companies that provide services in health and fitness usually will act as their own middlemen because they and their staff know their own programs and services better than anyone else does. Why have someone else retail (sell) it for you? Also, the customer pays a lower price when services are purchased directly from you.

Price Structures and Policies

Price structures and policies must be established carefully and in conjunction with sales tactics and distribution procedures. The price of a program or service will be affected by its development costs, how it will be distributed, the desired profit margin, competitors' prices, and how it will be sold. Your prices must be competitive to penetrate a market, to maintain or improve your market position, and then still to produce a profit.

Pricing health and fitness services should be based on the "four Cs": Consumers (target market or audience); Costs (resources, product development, labor, and suppliers); Competition (competitors' current market share and position); and Controls (company, government, or public policies and legislation).

Pricing must also be done strategically to guarantee that both the company and the client will be satisfied with what is being provided for the money. Following are six strategic pricing factors that you should consider.

- Compete on a nonprice basis (*nonprice competition*) while maintaining a profit margin. Provide more value for the dollar by giving more program for the money and providing better follow-up service.
- Price competitively if the company cannot compete on a nonprice basis. *Competitive pricing* is based on program availability and demand, and it often leads to service providers offering similar prices. However, if you can differentiate your programs and services from competitors, you may be able to price them slightly higher as they would have a different perceived value (Mulvihill & Konopa, 1986; Settle & Alreck, 1986). Eventually you can lower your prices if you want. This is called a "skimming" strategy (see Assael, 1985). This is interesting as many companies believe that lower initial prices will help them penetrate the market better. This is called a penetration pricing strategy (see Assael, 1985). On the other hand, consumers may perceive low prices as reflecting low quality. There will always be a relationship between the image you create for your services and the prices you charge for them.
- Charge separately for extras. Provide the client with a basic package and price, identify the possible extra services that may be purchased, and charge for these services. Do not include everything in one package and at one price because the cost may become prohibitive. Also, you will not be getting a fair and equitable price for the programs or services you are providing.
- Include provisions in the sales contract for price escalations and reductions. This is important if you are providing services over an extended period of time or if more clients will be using the service in the future. Clients will appreciate the fact that possible price changes were identified at the time of sale.
- Use consumers to help establish price schedules. This can be done through market research, investigating consumer acceptance of your competitors' pricing schedules, or simply identifying the price that creates the most purchasing. Although this will require some extra work, it is well worth your effort as proper pricing will lead to more sales and usually greater profits.

- Finally, when developing pricing structures and policies, you must consider methods of payment. A company does not want to price itself out of the market at either end of the spectrum, nor does it want its payment terms to do the same. One of the best ways to establish payment terms is to identify the pricing and payment trends in the health and fitness industry over the last 3 to 5 years and then compare your policies to the industry trend. Most payments are made on a cash or credit basis either immediately or within 30 days of receipt of an invoice. Payment policies must complement your pricing structures to achieve your sales goals.

The next section of the marketing analysis is advertising and promotion.

Advertising and Promotion

Advertising channels include print, radio, and television. Types of *promotion* include free product or service giveaways, free speeches, public appearances, membership in civic and professional associations, and sponsoring events such as races or aerobics contests. These examples will show you many methods you can use to advertise and promote a health and fitness business. These must be specified briefly in this section of the plan.

You may also want to discuss methods of initial client contact—such as personal sales, direct mail, or telemarketing—and the cost of developing the advertising and promotional campaign. You do not need to develop an advertising *budget* at this time. But be aware that the advertising budget should not be determined as a percentage of sales. Advertising expenditures should generate, not be a result of, revenue. You cannot allocate $1,000 for advertising and expect it to generate $1,000,000 worth of revenue. That is unrealistic. But you can determine from previous experience that $50,000 for advertising will result in $500,000 worth of revenue. Simply track how your clients or club members heard of your services, what prompted them to purchase them, and how much revenue these purchases brought in.

The market analysis is now complete. As you write your own business plan, you will see how the market and company and industry analyses influence your marketing decisions as well as decisions about strategy, management, and financial considerations, which will be discussed in chapter 3.

Chapter 3

Completing the Business Plan_____

Three analyses are discussed in this chapter: strategic, management, and financial. The analyses correlate in describing how you will maintain and market your services, facilities, products, or programs; who will be responsible for each segment of this operational process; and how much it should cost to continue and/or expand your business operations. A sample business plan for a health and fitness program *provider* is presented to illustrate how each segment of a business plan must be tailored to fit a specific business and its market.

The Strategic Analysis

The *strategic analysis* includes action plans for implementing your company's or your program's goals and objectives; strategies and tactics, which specify the steps included in the action plan; key *performance indicators*, which measure progress in attaining goals; project completion schedules, which measure milestones of achievement in the process of attaining each goal; operating assumptions, which define the expected conditions under which your company will operate; strategic opportunities which your company will use to build on its strengths in a given market; and strategic obstacles, which are problems that pose a challenge but can be resolved.

The strategic analysis is the blueprint for success that your business must follow to gain a substantial market share in the health and fitness industry. It also can serve as the foundation for a more sophisticated process known as strategic planning, which is the long-range planning a company should do for all its business ventures (Gardner, Rachlin, & Sweeny, 1986; Hamermesh, 1986; Marrus, 1984; *Optimal Health*, 1987; Steiner, 1979).

Action Plans

You must pay close attention to the action plans that will be developed so that market potentials can be maximized with a minimum of risk. This means that the entire plan of action must be specified completely, spelling out each step in detail. For example, assume that you are trying to convince your superiors of the importance of implementing a high blood pressure screening and follow-up program for the company's employees. Your plan of action may be as follows:

1. Gather information related to high blood pressure and its role as a risk factor in heart disease and stroke.
2. Provide cost/benefit data relative to high blood pressure and the possible savings that can accrue from simply identifying at-risk individuals through a basic screening.
3. Present ideas for the follow-up educational program that will follow the screening.
4. Perform the screening and inform those with high blood pressure to see a physician; then tell them that you will be contacting them about the follow-up program.
5. Contact those individuals who have been identified as being at risk either through the mail, personally, or by telephone and give them a date and time that the follow-up program will begin.
6. Provide the follow-up program and keep detailed records of the participants' behaviors and blood pressure readings.
7. Give a presentation to company executives that shows the results of the program.

This brief plan of action is a step-by-step example to help you so that program risks can be minimized and potentials maximized. By adhering to detail in developing and implementing the strategic marketing plans, your company or programs will become more successful.

As discussed there are several components to the strategic analysis. Each one is equally important in developing this section of the business plan and to the future development of the marketing plan.

Goals and Objectives

Goals and objectives must be properly developed and described. Goal statements are qualitative and refer to what the business wants to achieve over a specified period of time, such as the next year or the next several years. An example of a program goal for a hospital-based health and fitness facility is "to provide selected health promotion programs to targeted segments of the community." The objective for this goal is a quantifiable statement about how the programs will be provided to the community.

Objectives are set over a short period of time because they identify the immediate result of an action. Objectives are specific, measurable, set within a reasonable time frame for achievement, moderately difficult to achieve, and concisely and clearly stated. A possible objective for the example goal stated above is "The wellness center will offer senior citizens two programs per month—The Myths of Aging, and Managing the Stress of Retirement—and will have at least 10 people attend each program." This objective can now serve as a foundation for the strategies that will help this hospital-based center achieve its goal.

Often a business owner will try to develop goals and objectives before writing the business plan. This is perfectly acceptable and is often recommended. It provides a foundation on which to build because the basic mission and philosophy of the company are clearly spelled out by the goals and objectives. Whether or not these are written before the plan or during it, goals and objectives must adhere to particular criteria to be functional.

As another example of a business goal and how several objectives are developed to support and reach that goal, assume that you have successfully provided a stress management program for the executives of your company. They were so pleased with it that they want you to market and sell it to other companies. Your goal might be to provide executive stress management programs for other companies in the area. Your objective could be to service a minimum of 10 companies each year at a cost of $1,000 per program. This will provide $10,000 per year in revenue.

Your plan of action to achieve this goal and objective is as follows:

1. Besides you, a minimum of one other staff person will be trained to sell and provide the executive stress management program. This training will be completed in 1 month.
2. Ten companies will be contacted each week in hope of obtaining two personal appointments with the company decision makers.
3. Each presentation will last no longer than 30 minutes and will include a description of the program's components, the benefits of the program, the costs, the return to the client, and the date the promotion begins.

Taking time to write your goal statement and objective and the actions required to achieve them will save you time because you already will have specified the terms of your plan.

Strategies and Tactics

Strategies are the conceptual procedures and programs by which the action plans will be organized to enable the company to achieve its goals and objectives (King, 1986). Strategies are closely related to tactics, which are the actual methods by which the strategies are implemented.

An example of a strategy is to use telemarketing to gain initial entry into a market. You have developed an exercise program for seniors that emphasizes flexibility training but still offers a moderate cardiovascular workout. You begin to market your program by telephoning condominium complexes, nursing homes, country clubs, and other locations that possess a large senior population. Another strategy associated with this market entry strategy is to price programs and services similar to competitors who already have programs in effect. The tactic involves offering clients more for their money, possibly by going to them rather than having them come to you. Perhaps the best way to view strategies and tactics is that a strategy is the thought or the decision-making process about what should be done and how, whereas a tactic is the behavioral implementation of that thought process.

Some questions must be answered when determining strategies and tactics (King, 1986). First, what are the assumptions that your company has made with respect to devising the strategies and their associated tactics? Assumptions refer to beliefs that you accept as true without questioning them, such as that health and fitness programs can be profitable. Second, what are the preferred and alternative courses of action that will enable your company to achieve its goals and objectives of making these programs profitable? Third, what resources are necessary to achieve the desired results? This refers to finances, staff, programs, and anything related to achieving results. Fourth, what are the risks/rewards or costs/benefits of any or all of the strategies? Finally, who will be responsible for implementing each strategy and held accountable for its results? Are you, as the program director, solely responsible for everything, or will portions of the implementation process be assigned to others?

Strategies are based on your marketing goals, your target markets, the industry life cycle, and your competitive position. Implementing these plans will direct the company toward its goals and objectives. A well-written section on strategies will help identify the key performance indicators that help determine whether your company will be successful.

Key Performance Indicators

These are the criterion measures, both financial and otherwise, that your company will use to track and evaluate its progress toward its goals. Some of these indicators include sales revenue, market share, profitability, advertising and promotion costs, costs per lead, the numbers of participants per program, and sales calls. Other indicators are the number of direct inquiries you receive for every advertisement you run and requests for additional information about the programs.

Project Completion Schedule

This schedule (see Project Completion Schedule form) charts the milestones to be achieved, their deadlines for achievement, and who, if anyone, is responsible for completing each project. If the entire strategic analysis section is the map for success, then this subsection is the legend. It gives the reader all the necessary information at a glance. The schedule demonstrates the company's ability to plan systematically for goal attainment in an organized and timely manner as well as its ability to minimize the risks involved by clearly defining each project.

The project completion schedule is also called an activity schedule or a project schedule. Regardless of its name its function is to provide a graphic timeline of what your company expects to do and when. To complete this form, write the name of the project in the first column and mark off the completion dates of each activity across the schedule. Another column can be added to identify the person assigned to oversee the project. You can then compare the completion dates of any business activity with the projected dates from the schedule.

Operating Assumptions

These are the expected external conditions under which your company will operate. You must identify the conditions that are most important to the health and fitness industry as well as the trends that are likely to occur during the time frame of the business plan. A guide to determining the operating assumptions of a company is to categorize the assumptions as economical (overall growth, inflation price trends, and service costs); industrial (growth rates, new products and services development, changes in program distribution patterns, changes in consumer behavior such as buying desires or capabilities, and changes in competitor's behavior); and outside influences (regulatory agencies and suppliers and vendors). Other assumptions that may also be relevant to the business should be specified. These may include the availability of programs, the staff to implement those programs, and the availability of financial resources to continue advertising the programs. You need to be specific in determining the assumptions under which your company or program will operate.

Strategic Opportunities

These are the opportunities that your company will expand on to use its strengths in gaining a better market position. For example, your nearest competitor will provide smoking cessation programs to companies only if the companies agree to repeat the programs four times a year. This may not be exactly what the client wants. But you on the other hand can provide smoking cessation programs whenever they are needed, and you

Project completion schedule

Project	JAN	FEB	MAR	APR	MAY	JUN	JUL	AUG	SEP	OCT	NOV	DEC	JAN	FEB	MAR	APR	MAY	JUN	JUL	AUG	SEP	OCT	NOV	DEC

will even contract with a client for single programs. This is an excellent way to develop a client base and start to earn your share of the market. You will have found an opportunity in what appeared to be a competitor's strength. So it is obvious that a comprehensive identification of strategic opportunities will enable your company to more accurately determine its marketing strategies and tactics.

Strategic Obstacles

Strategic obstacles are those problems that currently exist but that cannot be resolved within the life span of the business plan nor the strategy implementation process. Remember that the life span of the plan may be 1, 3, or 5 years, and of the tactical plans only weeks or months. You must identify the obstacles that cannot be overcome during the plan's time frame. Some of these may be a lack of advertising capital to gain a significant portion of a desired market, too many program providers in the low to moderate-price range, and not enough programs to offer clients a wide variety of services. The important point is to not ignore these obstacles but to identify them and then eventually develop a plan of action (strategies and tactics) by which to overcome them.

In the health and fitness industry, various types of strategies can be developed depending on whether the setting is corporate (Chenoweth, 1987; Kizer, 1987; O'Donnell & Ainsworth, 1984; Opatz, 1985, 1987; Parkinson, 1982), commercial/private (Ardell & Tager, 1982; Bellingham & Tager, 1986; Gerson, 1987; Patton, Grantham, Gerson, & Gettman, 1986, 1989) or hospital based (Clair, 1987; Sol, 1987). Identify your setting and the strategies and tactics that are appropriate for it.

This completes the strategic analysis section, which, in its simplest form, is really a set of behavioral action plans. They detail how goals will be achieved and who will be responsible for achieving them. The management analysis section which follows will describe the people and skills and characteristics they need to carry out these plans.

The Management Analysis

The *management analysis* is a detailed description of all the key personnel in the organization. The first part of this section identifies the management positions within the company and the people who will fill those positions. The simplest way to identify the positions and the people is to specify the position title followed by a brief job description and then to write a short biography of the person who will fill that position. You could also use the person's résumé. An example of a job description for an executive director follows.

Job Description: **Executive Director**

Qualifications

1. Doctoral degree (Ph.D. or Ed.D.)
2. Minimum of 2–5 years experience as director (manager, supervisor) of a spa, health club, or fitness facility
3. Knowledge and experience in development and implementation of health promotion programs
4. Knowledge of budget preparation, revenue projection, financial review, and personnel management
5. American College of Sports Medicine certification as health fitness director or program director.

Responsibilities

1. Report directly to vice president
2. Develop and supervise all operations, programs, and personnel
3. Hire and train staff in all areas
4. Develop yearly budget
5. Conduct montly and yearly financial reviews
6. Develop public relations and marketing stategies
7. Conduct ongoing training workshops for staff
8. Conduct department head meetings
9. Conduct employee evaluation interviews
10. Develop departmental performance standards

A job description for a fitness coordinator also lists qualifications and responsibilities.

Job description: **Fitness Coordinator**

Qualifications

1. Masters degree in physical education, exercise physiology, or related field.
2. Minimum 1 year of supervisory experience of a fitness staff in either a spa, health club, or fitness facility

3. Knowledge of administrative procedures and personnel management
4. Background in health promotion (specifically, stress management), nutritional awareness, and lifetime fitness
5. American College of Sports Medicine Certification as health fitness instructor

Responsibilities

1. Report to executive director
2. Supervise operations of fitness center
3. Supervise all department heads
4. Develop fitness evaluation tests and protocols
5. Develop exercise prescriptions and programs
6. Develop counseling procedures
7. Hire and train fitness staff
8. Conduct departmental meetings
9. Conduct employee evaluation interviews
10. Conduct ongoing training workshops for staff

A second job description method is similar except that the résumés are placed in an appendix to the business plan. Whichever method is chosen, a management analysis requires that the first position described be the president or chief executive officer. It can also begin with the program director if the plan is being written for a department that serves as its own business unit. Then proceed to describe all the other important positions.

Once you choose the method of describing the management team, describe the structural relationships among the positions. The example in Figure 3.1 is a standard, top-down organizational chart. Using an organizational chart to describe your management structure makes relationships clear to members of your team.

Personnel Pro Forma

The management analysis seeks to identify the important personnel within the organization. However, all company or departmental staffing requirements are not achieved at one time. More often than not, a company must grow into its full complement of staff members. This is especially true in the health and fitness industry, whether the organization is a club, hospital, or private or corporate center. A personnel *pro forma* should therefore be developed to specify future manpower needs. The personnel pro forma lists all the expected job positions and then identifies when

Sample organizational chart, Department of Health Promotion

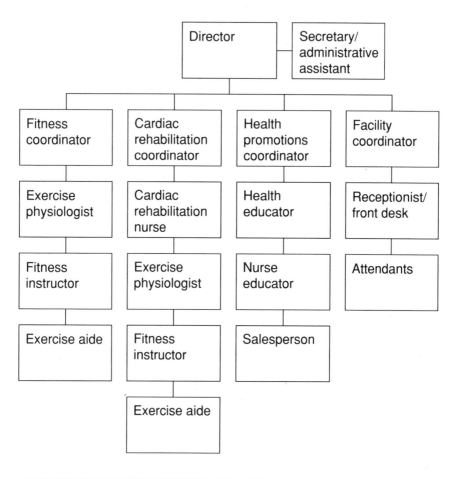

Figure 3.1.   Sample organizational chart for a health promotion department.

they will be opened. The Health Club Personnel Pro Forma is an example of a basic personnel pro forma.

Management Philosophy

This section of the management analysis outlines the intended management philosophy of the company or the department. There are countless management theories that have been developed over the years, some of

Health Club Personnel Pro Forma

Job category	19___	19___	19___	19___
Administrative and general				
President/owner				
Executive director				
Secretary/bookkeeper				
Receptionist				
Total				
Fitness				
Fitness coordinator				
Exercise physiologist				
Exercise Instructor				
Aerobics instructor				
Other				
Total				
Marketing and sales				
Sales/marketing director				
Sales personnel				
Total				
Total personnel				

which are still in use while others are outdated. Whichever philosophy you select, it is instructive for corporate executives and department heads within a company to describe how they plan to operate their company. This will benefit all personnel as they will know what to expect in any given situation.

The Financial Analysis

The last section of the business plan is the *financial analysis*, which must be consistent with all the other parts of the plan. The financial analysis serves several purposes in the business plan.

- It helps the company prepare an operating budget for all its departmental areas as well as helping departments prepare their own operating budgets.
- It identifies business income potential and projected expenses.
- It identifies *capital* needs, such as the amount of money needed to purchase equipment or programs or simply to start the operation.
- It allows for financial *forecasting* based on the pro forma income statement.
- It allows for the preparation of a *balance sheet* that lists company assets, liabilities, and equity.
- It helps the company and each revenue-producing department prepare a *cash-flow statement*.
- It tells creditors and investors that the company is solvent and what it expects to achieve financially (see Crego, Deaton, & Schiffrin, 1986; Leza & Placenia, 1982).

Financial Schedules

The financial analysis consists of four main financial schedules: an income statement, a balance sheet, a cash-flow statement, and a budget. There should also be additional schedules in the financial plan such as departmental budgets, a *break-even analysis*, a *profit-and-loss statement*, and financial performance statistics (cf. Cohen, 1987; Crego et al., 1986).

It is recommended that the finance department of the company, or whomever is responsible for the financial operations of the company or department, be capable of preparing all these schedules monthly, quarterly, and annually. This will provide both an ongoing view and a record of the financial status of the company and will also provide figures for future performance comparisons.

Many individuals in the health and fitness industry may not be familiar with financial terms and ratios. Therefore, a brief definition and description will be provided for the major financial schedules that must be included in a business plan. Sample forms are also provided for each type of financial schedule. Additionally, the glossary at the back of the book lists definitions of some of the more important *financial ratios* that you will encounter while operating your business. More detailed descriptions can be found in several good college texts on finance as well as in Caro (1986), Cohen (1987), O'Donnell and Ainsworth (1984), and Patton et al (1989).

Pro Forma. A pro forma is simply a projection. A projection is an expectation of what will be or what will happen. The personnel pro forma was mentioned in the previous section as a projection of staffing needs. Financial pro formas are usually an income or expense statement, a balance sheet, or a cash-flow statement and project budget. Their purpose is to estimate/project expected costs and revenues. Examples of all these pro formas will be provided as they are mentioned.

Income Statement. The income statement describes the relationship among the company's revenues, expenses, and subsequent profit and loss over a given time period (see Table 3.1 on page 38). This period may be a month, a quarter, a year, a few years, or any length of time. Income statements should be prepared at least quarterly and definitely on an annual basis.

An income statement should always have two parts. The first reflects the operating transactions, or the money transferred between the buyer and your company as the provider of services. These operating transactions are placed on the income statement to depict quarterly summaries and then a yearly total. The second part of the income statement shows the total amounts as a percentage of sales, or the cost of goods sold. It is important to know exactly how much it costs your company to earn the revenue for a given product and how much of that revenue is actual profit.

Balance Sheet. The balance sheet lists all the company's assets and liabilities plus the owner's equity (see Table 3.2 on page 39). The balance sheet depicts the status of the company by identifying the relationship between the assets and the liabilities on any given date, not for a specified length of time. Assets are what a company owns, whereas liabilities are what it owes. Equity refers to assets that are above and beyond the liabilities.

Cash-Flow Statement. The cash-flow statement form identifies whether a company has sufficient cash available to honor its commitments and obligations (see the Pro Forma Monthly Cash-Flow Statement form on page 40). The statement helps the company determine if it will be in a positive cash-flow position (money is available) or in a negative, or deficit, cash-flow position (money is not being earned as rapidly as necessary).

This knowledge of cash-flow position can be used to determine whether the company needs to secure funds from creditors or investors or if the company has *liquidity*, meaning that it has money available and can use the excess capital to somehow improve its market position. Basically, the

Table 3.1 Pro Forma Income Statement
For the Fiscal Year _____ , 19___ , to _____ , 19___

	Quarter 1 2 3 4	Total Amount	% Sales
Revenue			
Gross sales		_____	_____
Less returns and allowances		_____	_____
Net sales		_____	_____
Cost of sales			
Beginning inventory		_____	_____
Cost of program production		_____	_____
Less ending inventory		_____	_____
Total cost of sales		_____	_____
Gross profit		_____	_____
Operating expenses			
Salaries and wages		_____	_____
Commissions		_____	_____
Employee benefits		_____	_____
Insurance		_____	_____
Rent		_____	_____
Depreciation		_____	_____
Interest payments		_____	_____
Other		_____	_____
Total operating expenses		_____	_____
Other expenses		_____	_____
Net income before taxes		_____	_____
Net profit		_____	_____

cash-flow statement tells where the money is coming from, how it is being used, and how much is actually necessary for the effective operation of the company.

Budget.   The budget is one of the most important schedules that can be included in the financial analysis section of the business plan (see Table 3.3 on page 41). It is often written first because it provides a guide for all the other schedules to follow. A budget is a companywide or departmental estimate of operating revenues and expenditures. These statements are usually prepared on an annual basis, and they are presented

Table 3.2 Pro Forma Balance Sheet
19 ___

Assets		Liabilities	
Current		**Current**	
Cash	___	Accounts payable	___
Accounts receivable		Short-term notes	___
less allowance for		Current portion of	
doubtful accounts	___	long-term notes	___
Net accounts receivable	___	Interest payable	___
Inventory	___	Taxes payable	___
Investments (shortterm)	___	Accrued payroll	___
Prepaid expenses	___	Total current liabilities	___
Long-term investments	___	**Long-term investments**	___
Fixed		**Equity**	
Land	___	Owner's	___
Buildings		or	
(less depreciation)	___	Partner's	___
Equipment		Total partner's equity	___
(less depreciation)	___	Shareholder's equity	___
Furniture		Stock (if any)	___
(less depreciation)	___		
Total net fixed assets	___		
Other assets	___		
Total assets	___	Total liabilities	
		and equity	___

Pro Forma Monthly Cash-Flow Statement
for the first 5 months fiscal year _____, 19___, to _____, 19___

	January	February	March	April	May
Receipts					
Cash sales					
Credit sales					
Loans					
Other					
Total receipts					
Disbursements					
Salaries					
Wages					
Benefits					
Materials					
Equipment					
Rent					
Insurance					
Advertising					
Taxes					
Loan payments					
Depreciation					
Total disbursements					
Total cash flow					
Beginning balance					
Ending balance					

Table 3.3 Health and Fitness Center Budget*

Item	Jan	Feb	Mar	Apr	May	June	July	Aug	Sept	Oct	Nov	Dec	Total	Variance
Revenues														
Memberships	40	40	40	40	40	40	40	40	40	40	40	40	480	
Assessments	8.33	8.33	8.33	8.33	8.33	8.33	8.33	8.33	8.33	8.33	8.33	8.33	100	
Health promotion	4.17	4.17	4.17	4.17	4.17	4.17	4.17	4.17	4.17	4.17	4.17	4.17	50	
Miscellaneous	.833	.833	.833	.833	.833	.833	.833	.833	.833	.833	.833	.833	10	
Total													640	
Expenses														
Salaries	15	15	15	15	15	15	15	15	15	15	15	15	180	
Benefits	3	3	3	3	3	3	3	3	3	3	3	3	36	
Equipment	10	10	10	10	10	10	10	10	10	10	10	10	120	
Supplies	1	1	1	1	1	1	1	1	1	1	1	1	12	
Marketing	2	2	2	2	2	2	2	2	2	2	2	2	24	
Advertising	4	4	4	4	4	4	4	4	4	4	4	4	48	
Utilities	2	2	2	2	2	2	2	2	2	2	2	2	24	
Rent	10	10	10	10	10	10	10	10	10	10	10	10	120	
Insurance	3	3	3	3	3	3	3	3	3	3	3	3	36	
Dues and subscriptions	.1	.1	.1	.1	.1	.1	.1	.1	.1	.1	.1	.1	1.2	
Meetings	.6	.6	.6	.6	.6	.6	.6	.6	.6	.6	.6	.6	7.2	
Miscellaneous	.5	.5	.5	.5	.5	.5	.5	.5	.5	.5	.5	.5	6	
Total													614.4	

*Budget in thousands

either for the entire year or broken down month by month. Budgets can also be developed on a monthly, quarterly, or multiannual basis.

The budget's purpose is to serve as a guide for the company or department as it carries out its daily activities. Everyone working for a health and fitness company should be aware whether they or their department are exceeding or operating within the budgetary limits.

It is recommended that all budgets contain a variance column. Variance is the percentage difference between the budget projections and the actual money spent or received. Expense lines in a budget should have a negative variance, which means that less money was spent than expected. Income lines should show a positive variance, which means that more money was made than was budgeted.

The variance also serves as a guide to determine whether financial controls are necessary for the coming year. This is where the profit-and-loss statement comes in. This statement is a monthly accounting of revenues and expenses in relation to the projected budget and the appropriate variances. The profit-and-loss statement looks just like the budget and has columns so that all the line items can be compared.

Break-Even Analysis.   The break-even analysis is used to evaluate the relationship among revenues and fixed and variable costs. Revenues are those monies that you earn from sales; fixed costs refer to those costs such as rent, utilities, telephone, and research and development that you would have to pay regardless of whether you sold a service or program; and variable costs are those costs such as payroll, advertising, production, and packaging of the product that change according to the number of programs that are sold (Caro, 1986). The break-even point is the point at which the revenues from sales cover all the costs associated with developing, producing, and selling the products or programs. Falling below this point means that you are losing money whereas rising above it means you are making a profit.

The break-even point tells you how many sales must be made to make a profit, how much profit you will make at a given level of sales, how your price structure and changes in it will affect profitability, and how cost increases or reductions will affect profitability (Cohen, 1987). You can determine the break-even point for any sales product simply by subtracting the variable cost from the price of the product, multiplying that by the sales volume or revenue, and then subtracting the fixed cost from that total. If the result is positive, you are making a profit. If it is negative, you are losing money. If the result is zero, you are breaking even.

For example, you decide to sell health risk appraisals to local corporations and need to conduct a break-even analysis for a 12-month period. You have determined that your fixed costs over that year will be $3,000 and your variable costs $5 per health risk appraisal, which does not include the fee that you charge the client. The fee for the health risk appraisal is $10 per test. To find your break-even point or, in this case, the number of health risk appraisals that you must sell, you simply plug the numbers into the formula described above to get a result of zero. Your break-even calculation would be as follows:

$$0 = 3,000 \div (10—5), \text{ or } 3,000 \div 5 = 600$$

$$600 \div 12 = 50$$

You need to sell 600 health risk appraisals to break even for the year, or 50 per month. A break-even analysis is illustrated in Figure 3.2.

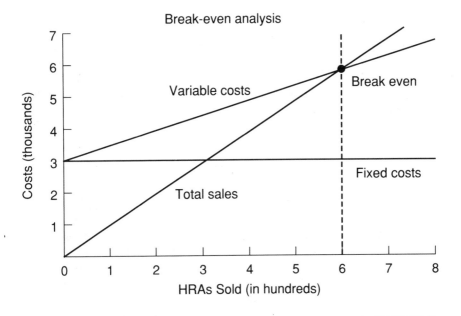

Figure 3.2. Break-even analysis for health risk assessment sales. HRA sales are indicated in hundreds.

The financial analysis section is now complete. It must coincide with all the other parts of the business plan. If there is a poor match—for example, the strategies and tactics that will be used to penetrate the market are not sufficiently powerful to create the revenues or cover the expenses that are identified in the pro formas—then both sections should be revised. The expected revenues and expenses must support the company's goals, objectives, and operating plans.

The business plan is also complete. It should be used as an ongoing management tool, and the business plan should be carried out in a dynamic manner. The factors that will affect your company's performance are now apparent. Business strategies and tactics must be implemented as they were outlined, but they must also be revised and updated as the industry changes and grows. Flexibility and creativity must be maintained in the plan so that all actions, even those that have been modified, will lead to success. The business plan must always be used as a working document to guide the company or department toward achieving stated goals and objectives.

A Sample Business Plan

Now let's pull together all the things you have learned so far by applying them in an abbreviated business plan written for a fictitious company, AAA Fitness, Inc., a health promotion program provider. The plan will follow the outline for a standard business plan that was presented in chapter 2. Use this plan only as a guide. Some of the material may be pertinent to your situation, and some may not. The purpose of providing this sample plan is to show you how the components of a business plan are coordinated into a working document.

Executive Summary

AAA Fitness provides exercise and health promotion programs to clients who do not have the staff expertise to do so on their own. This plan describes the company in detail, the type of services it provides, where and how it intends to do its business, who the key people are in the company, and the financial requirements and conditions under which the company must operate.

The company is a for-profit division of a larger hospital health promotion department that provides programs to the community and to small and mid-sized corporations. AAA Fitness was formed to service those companies with less than 100 employees and to attempt to group several companies together to take advantage of program offerings. The staff of AAA consists of a coordinator and a health and fitness specialist/salesperson. The company is capable of networking with many other professionals in the health and fitness business as well as other departments in the hospital whenever the need may arise.

Several factors, including the lack of competition in the market and the support of the hospital, allow AAA to set a series of ascending business and financial goals. The original business goals are simple. First, the company wants to establish itself as a service provider in the health and fitness field. It will do so through publicity exposure and a minimal amount of print advertising, direct mail, personal contact, and telephone contact. Second, the company wants to secure enough accounts in each of its first 3 years of existence so that net profits are at least 15% of revenue. Third, the company wants to establish a reputation for providing better follow-up service for its clients than any competitors in its geographic service area.

Company Analysis

The strengths of the company include its personnel—who not only studied the areas of health and fitness throughout school but also continue to live the lifestyle as role models—the apparent lack of competition, and the uniqueness of offering health promotion programs to small- and medium-sized businesses. Few of these companies even considered providing such programs to their employees.

Some of the company's weaknesses include a lack of a major advertising campaign, a small staff, a small geographic service area, and a lack of knowledge about the benefits of employee fitness on the part of prospective customers. The latter two weaknesses can be viewed as opportunities because the clients know that the person calling on them to sell the programs will also present the programs. This helps maintain constant contact between the company representative and the client. Also, the lack of knowledge on the part of the public is really a challenge for AAA to educate the clients as to their needs and to the benefits of health and fitness programs.

The only threat that exists is that some area hospitals are beginning to investigate the possibility of starting their own health promotion programs. These include programs in stress management, smoking cessation, weight control, and employee exercise. It is difficult for a small, for-profit company to compete with these nonprofit hospitals. Another threat arises from the proliferation of new consulting firms that are entering the market to offer similar programs.

Company History

The history of AAA Fitness is very brief. It was formed as an outgrowth of a hospital health promotion department whose administrator decided that there was a market for a for-profit entity to provide health and fitness programs to small- and medium-sized companies. The fitness company was formed with a minimal staff to inaugurate its activities. Each staff member has clearly described responsibilities, and the other departments in the hospital can be counted on to provide whatever support is needed.

Program and Service Offerings

Since AAA Fitness is a small company, it was decided to keep its program and service offerings specific. This was primarily due to the staff's areas of specialization and its ability to deliver a certain amount of programs in a given time frame. The initial program offerings will be stress management, weight control, and aerobics.

Prospective Markets and Clients

The primary market for AAA Fitness is businesses with fewer than 100 employees in a geographic service area of 5 miles from the company's downtown office. The secondary market includes businesses of similar sizes within a 10-mile radius. A third market area, but one that will not be actively sought, is community and religious groups within the service radius of 5 to 10 miles. This last group of potential clients will be serviced on a referral-only basis.

Technology and Resources

The technology of AAA is current in that it uses a computer to track its clients and process data and uses the telephone for much of its marketing activity. The resources of the company are considerable as it can draw on hospital personnel as the need arises.

Major Competitors and Competitive Position

The major competitors to AAA are nonprofit hospitals offering community health and fitness programs at no charge and several private consulting practices. Although these groups are the major competitors of AAA, the competitive size of the industry is still rather limited. Because the company cannot determine any type of competitive position, it will create its niche in the local market first. If that is successful, then AAA will expand its market to include some city- and statewide programs.

Success Factors

The success factors for AAA Fitness include signing one new client every 2 to 3 months, developing a positive reputation and image in the business and health and fitness communities, and achieving revenues of $75,000 the first year to meet the goal of securing net profits that equal 15% of the revenue for each of the first 3 years.

Cost Comparisons

AAA Fitness decided that its program costs will be based on a sliding scale according to the number of participants and that a 15% profit margin will be built directly into the cost. These costs are also similar to those being charged by competitors (when there are charges), so clients need to choose services based on perceived quality. AAA wants to make its price schedule cost competitive and within the limits that the market can afford.

Industry Analysis

The health and fitness industry can be defined as very large in scope as there are service providers, equipment manufacturers, and facility designers. AAA Fitness will specialize in the service aspect of health and fitness although many providers of health and fitness programs already exist. Therefore, AAA will focus on three primary programs: stress management, weight control, and exercise programs.

Growth Rate

The growth rate of the health and fitness industry is rapid. This is shown in the results of surveys completed by the International Racquet Sports Association (IRSA) and other professional and recreational groups that conclude that more people are engaging in some form of physical activity and that more businesses are providing programs for their employees than in the past.

Key Growth Factors

The key growth factors for the health and fitness industry revolve around the desire to look and feel better, to lead healthier lifestyles, and to live longer. This has not only involved more people in health and fitness activities, but it has sent people looking for reliable sources of information. In response, hospitals and private consulting firms have begun to provide services and programs. The consumer's desire to purchase quality health and fitness programs and the increasing acceptance of health promotion programs in the workplace signify that the industry is strong and continues to grow.

Financial Operating Characteristics

For the most part, the health and fitness industry operates as does any typical business. Providers accept cash, check, or credit cards as payment for their services, and AAA Fitness will be no exception. The company will either accept half the payment prior to the start of a program and the other half on completion or bill a client for the total amount on completion of the program. All invoices require that payment be made within 30 days. However, the company wants to remain flexible with clients regarding their ability to pay. This is one way the company can maintain a reputation as being service oriented.

Industry Life Cycle

The increasing number of people engaging in health and fitness activities, the number of companies entering the consulting field, and the number of corporations beginning to offer employee programs show that the health and fitness industry is only beginning the growth stage of its life cycle. This makes many competitive strategies available to AAA, such as introducing new programs, developing more flexible pricing strategies, and upgrading, or offering current clients newer or better services. Because the industry is in the growth stage, the chances are high that AAA will continue to grow and become more successful.

Market Analysis

The scope of the market that AAA has chosen to service includes small- and medium-sized businesses within a radius of 5 to 10 miles of its office location. Further expansion will be considered at a later date as the company becomes more successful.

Market Segmentation

The market is segmented geographically by the chosen scope, and the clients are segmented by the number of people they employ. Typical demographics and other segmentation procedures are not necessary at this time.

Market Barriers

AAA does not experience any barriers to market entry as it is an offshoot of a hospital program and clients are already attracted to the hospital's other health care services.

Market Demand and Market Share

The demand for programs and services that AAA provides is constantly increasing, and it is expected that the market share will also increase. Even so, the market share will always be small because of the selected service area. This will be especially true if the calculations were based on national statistics, in which case the market share will always be less than 1%. If the calculations were based on the number of AAA program users in relation to the total number of potential users, the numbers might increase to about 5%. These percentages are acceptable to hospital administration and management as a 5%, market share all but guarantees profitability.

Market Sales

The desired amount of market sales for AAA Fitness in its first year of operation is $75,000. This will be achieved by obtaining at least six new clients during the fiscal year, requesting two referrals from each of these clients, continuing to service current hospital clients, and providing follow-up service to accounts that are completed.

Sales Tactics and Distribution Channels

The sales program will be performed simply. The company representative will develop a prospect list from personal contacts and resource books. These prospects will be qualified and then individually contacted. A personal meeting will be scheduled so that the prospect and the AAA representative can determine how a specific program will best meet the client's needs. Personal selling is the only method AAA will utilize. The same is true for the distribution of the programs. The representative who makes the sale is responsible for supplying the client with the program and the follow-up service. Again, this is done personally, and all contacts are to be followed with a confirmation letter.

Price Structures and Policies

The price structures and policies are developed after a careful analysis of the competition. AAA will price its programs and services to reflect coverage of all costs including development and implementation, remain competitive, and then maintain a 15% profit margin. The payment methods are cash, credit card, or check, and payments either are made immediately or clients are invoiced for services performed.

Advertising and Promotion

The advertising and promotional campaigns will remain simple and inexpensive. Business cards, brochures, personal appearances, and attendance at community functions will be used to develop the company's public image. There will also be a minimal amount of print advertising to provide name recognition for the new company. The goal of the advertising and promotional campaigns is to enable AAA Fitness to receive most of its subsequent business through referrals from satisfied customers.

Other promotional efforts will involve performing charitable work within the community such as speaking before civic groups or working with non-profit organizations. The result will be image enhancement and self-referrals from interested consumers. These minimal advertising efforts are considered sufficient to help the company achieve its goals.

Strategic Analysis

This section will describe the goals and objectives, key performance indicators, and operating costs of AAA Fitness, Inc.

Goals and Objectives

The primary business goal for AAA Fitness is to obtain one new client every 2 to 3 months. The second goal is to achieve gross revenues of $75,000 for the year. The third business goal is to develop new programs or to custom design programs for clients. This will be accomplished through research of program content and of the company's professional network. The overall objective of these goals is for the company to become more well known in the health and fitness industry as a leader in the provision of quality programs and services.

Key Performance Indicators

The key performance indicators are easily specified. The first is obtaining gross revenues of $75,000 with a minimum 10% increase during each of the next 5 years. The second indicator is signing six new clients each year. The third indicator is maintaining a profit margin of at least 15% on programs and services provided to clients. The final key performance indicator is the receipt of positive feedback and complete client satisfaction relative to the programs that are or will be provided.

Operating Assumptions

There are only a few assumptions under which AAA expects to operate. One assumption is that the clients agree to pay cash for the services provided either on an invoice basis or on completion of the program. Another assumption is that the entry of new competitors into the market will not much affect AAA as most of its new business will, hopefully, come from referrals. Finally, AAA Fitness is capable of providing programs at company sites or central locations. The only strategic obstacle to any of the services AAA will provide is that the company might overextend itself by contracting with more clients than the staff can handle.

Management Analysis

The company consists of two key staff members—a coordinator with a master's degree in exercise physiology and health promotion and a health and fitness specialist/salesperson with a bachelor's degree in adult fitness/health promotion. The management philosophy of AAA is to treat all employees (whether paid staff or contract persons) as professionals, to provide them with the responsibility to produce the best possible program for the clients, and to give them the latitude to inject their own personalities, thoughts, and feelings into the programs they provide.

Financial Analysis

Information on the financial analysis of AAA Fitness is unavailable because the company is fictitious. But you can review Table 3.3 on page 41 to see what the budget pro forma for this company might look like. Also, the income and expense pro formas are simply the separation of the revenue and expense sections of this budget. Finally, there is no balance sheet because the company has not yet conducted any business. You may wish to substitute your own company's balance sheet to get an idea of how to complete this section.

Chapter 4

The Marketing Plan

Before we begin to discuss the marketing plan, it is important to note the different types of services offered by health and fitness companies. These are activity, facility, and consultation services. In the health and fitness industry, service is the primary product. Companies do offer facilities and fitness products, but the owners and directors of these companies recognize that their success depends on providing good service, the key to customer satisfaction. Customer satisfaction is based on the perceived value of the service being offered and how well that service satisfies a specific customer need.

Marketing Activity Services

Activity services refer to the design, development, and implementation of exercise and health promotion programs in or for a company or organization (Patton et al., 1986). These programs may be already developed by your company, which has convinced a client to purchase them. Or you can custom tailor a particular program for a client to satisfy a specific need. In either case, the success of the activity being offered depends on your availability and flexibility as the provider.

Sometimes you, as the provider, can select the classes, the types of programs, and their presentation times. For example, you have a stress management program that meets weekly in a community center. You have informed several new clients of the meeting time and place. They must determine if the time, place, and course content are convenient and beneficial for them, especially as you are in control of the offering. There are other cases, however, in which clients will dictate exactly what they want. They will tell you which program they want, when they want it delivered, where it will be delivered, how long each session will be, and how often the group will meet. They are now in control. In either case, their level of satisfaction will determine whether the services contract is maintained or renewed.

Marketing Facility Services

The second service is the provision of a facility. Many hospitals, health and fitness centers, and YMCAs work closely with businesses to offer either programs or facilities to their employees. It would be ideal if every health and fitness provider had its own facility to offer to clients. Unfortunately, this is not the case. Only a few providers, such as hospital-based health and fitness centers, YMCAs, and some health clubs, have the capability of offering both service programs and exercise facilities to clients.

Even if you do not have the facility resources that clubs and hospitals have, you can still provide your clients with a facility. A service provider can work as a liaison between clients and facilities and get them to meet. Any exercise facility or health promotion program will welcome your efforts to provide them with new clients. Your personal compensation arrangements for acting in this capacity will need to be worked out with the host facility. The facility must get its fee, your clients must feel that they are getting value for the dollar, and you must feel that you have been fairly compensated. Then everybody wins.

Marketing Consultation Services

The third approach to providing services is to act strictly as a consultant. Consultants operate in many areas of the industry, including facility design, program development, staff recruitment and training, facility operations, and club or program management. Consultants also help clients write business and marketing plans and design marketing programs. When a company decides to go into the health and fitness business or to expand some part of an already existing business, it will often hire a consultant to help determine the feasibility of entering this area of business.

A consultant must be skilled in the areas in which the client has contracted for services. Consumers will purchase information from a consultant when they feel that the consultant can provide them with more and better information than they could get elsewhere. Remember that the information that the consumers purchase and that you are providing must enable them to reach their goals and satisfy their needs and desires. Otherwise your consulting services are not giving them what they paid for.

The type of service that a company will offer must be finalized before penetrating a new or existing market. Once the company decides on either activities, facilities, or consulting (which often is a combination of the first two services), it must determine the means of positioning the company and penetrating the market. Market positioning and penetration are the reasons for developing the marketing plan.

Writing the marketing plan involves gathering information in specific areas and then placing this material in the appropriate section of the plan. However, you must comprehend the concept of marketing before actually writing the plan.

Marketing is more than just sales, advertising, promotion, or *public relations*. Marketing has been defined as the exchange of activities (goods, products, programs, and services) conducted by individuals and organizations for the purpose of satisfying consumers' needs and achieving marketers' goals (Murphy & Enis, 1985). This definition simply means that two parties exchange an item voluntarily, usually at some cost, and both feel that they have benefited from the exchange.

Also, the exchange must take place through a channel of distribution (the marketplace) as a result of a communication process (advertising, promotion) that has taken place between the two parties. The simplest example of this process is when a client responds to your advertisement for a corporate stress management program, pays you to provide the program, and then you conduct it at an agreed-on site.

Companies view marketing as a means to help themselves and consumers obtain their respective objectives. Consumers often perceive marketing as something companies do to achieve corporate profits. On the other hand, consumers rely on marketing as the sole means of satisfying their own desires, needs, and wants. The match between the company's marketing program and the consumer's perceptions will determine whether and when the consumer will purchase the programs or services (Settle & Alreck, 1986).

From Your Business Plan to Your Marketing Plan

Marketing involves identifying and satisfying customer needs, developing new and maintaining existing programs or services, targeting and positioning these to specific consumer segments, developing a mix of strategies to influence consumer purchases, evaluating the environment and the effect of strategies and tactics, engaging in competition, and determining the success and failure of the chosen marketing approach (Assael, 1985; Bagozzi, 1986a, 1986b; Rapp & Collins, 1987).

The marketing plan describes how the company will engage in these activities, and it must be based on the market analysis section of the business plan. Unfortunately, many companies use this section as their marketing plan, but that is a mistake. The business plan describes the business and many nonmarketing activities such as program or product development, departmental budgets and personnel, and past company successes and failures. The marketing plan flows from the business plan and is not meant to replace or be replaced by it.

The major areas you need to address as you write your marketing plan include: market analysis, *competitive analysis*, target markets and entry strategies, market positioning techniques, marketing mix, and marketing strategies and tactics. As in your business plan, you should begin with an executive summary which will incude the description and rationale for the marketing plan; description of your program; projections of your sales and profits; and your current competitive position, market niche, and market share.

The Market Analysis

The market analysis section must include the same information that was provided in the business plan, including the results of the market research study and whether it is feasible to enter the market; an identification of the market scope, distribution procedures, and market entry and exit barriers; product/service demand within a market segment; potential market share; and sales projections. The analysis should also include an analysis of major competitors, their current market position and rank, and your current pricing strategy.

The market analysis helps identify whether the market is attractive enough for the company to do business in. *Market attractiveness* is based on whether the market is large enough to support your company's entry into it, its potential for growth, the number of customers in the market who are aware of and who can afford to pay for your services, the number of competitors in the market, the ease with which you can enter or exit the market, and the market's referral potential. Market attractiveness is an important factor in determining whether you should proceed with your plan.

You can further refine the market analysis process by responding to several questions posed by Marrus (1984).

• What market is the company in?

- How big is the market in terms of either the number of clients or dollar volume?
- What is the expected growth rate of the market in the next year or two?
- What stage of the life cycle is the market currently in?
- What are the key success factors for a company in this market?
- Is the market stable, or is it fluctuating?
- Are most competitors entering the market? Leaving the market?
- What is the primary basis of competition in the market? Price? Quality? Something else?

An outline of a comprehensive market analysis follows.

A Comprehensive Market Analysis Outline

I. Market Research

   A. Feasibility Study

   B. Needs Assessment

   C. Consumer Interest Survey

   D. Competitor Survey

II. Market Segmentation Procedures

   A. Demographics

   B. Geographic

   C. Psychographics

   D. Sociographics

III. Market Life Cycle

   A. Introduction

   B. Growth

   C. Maturity

   D. Decline

IV. Market Demand

   A. High Demand, High Supply

   B. High Demand, Low Supply

   C. Low Demand, High Supply

   D. Low Demand, Low Supply

By following this outline you will be able to address your market's particular characteristics.

The Competitive Analysis

Asking yourself the following questions will help you evaluate your service and market in relation to those of your competitors (Marrus, 1984).

- What is the company's present or desired market share?
- Who are the major competitors?
- What are their market shares?
- What are their strengths and weaknesses?
- How does your company compare to the competition on factors such as price, quality, service, and follow-up?
- What is the distinctive competence of your company, that is, the one thing it does better than anyone else?
- How does the company's financial status compare to that of the competition?
- What are the company and its competitors doing to ensure the future of the health and fitness industry?

To determine if a new service venture can be launched, combine the information from your answers to these questions with your data on market attractiveness. The information will be indispensable when you write your comprehensive competitive analysis. A comprehensive competitive analysis is used to help you make better marketing decisions and achieve the following goals:

- Accumulate current information about competitors and communicate this information to the staff for more effective decision making within your company.
- Draw application implications from your marketing information.
- Formulate competitive marketing strategies and tactics.
- Track short-term developments and long-term trends.
- Prepare an effective marketing program, complete with contingency plans.

Meeting these goals, particularly the goal of formulating competitive marketing strategies and tactics, will lead you to analyze and evaluate your competition. No matter how qualified your company is to provide services, it will not succeed unless you find out who your competitors are and how well they can compete. Information must be gathered to monitor the current competition, to identify their strengths and weaknesses, and to predict the entry of new competitors to the market.

Every company should develop a profile of its significant competitors. The first step is to realize that all competitors in a given market place share some common characteristics, including similar geographic service areas, suppliers, target markets, operating costs, and strategic marketing assumptions. Competitors will also use similar marketing mix strategies and implementation procedures. You can use the form on page 60 as you analyze your competitors.

After you analyze your competitors, you should analyze your own company's competitive ability again. This will help you draw accurate comparisons and contrasts and can make the difference between deciding to continue to pursue a given market and deciding to discontinue pursuit.

It is important to continue to gather and evaluate competitor information and compare your findings with information about your own company. Focus on your three major competitors, for they will have the greatest influence on your relative market share (Buzzell & Gale, 1987). An outline of competitor information sources follows on page 61.

Other sources of information include newspaper articles about the competition, trade shows and professional associations, suppliers and vendors, trade magazines, previous employees of competitors, related business and social contacts, customer service information, new product/program/service announcements, annual reports (called 10 Ks), and advertising and promotional campaigns.

After the information has been collected, the competitive profile must be further developed and refined according to critical marketing factors (Weinrauch, 1987). You must perform a SWOT analysis on each competitor using the chart shown in chapter 2 and determine the competitor's market share, position, rank, pricing policies, geographic service areas, customer follow-up, and plans for the future. This information will also help you determine the attractiveness of the target market because you will know how powerful your competitors are in that market. It can also help you decide on the type of service you wish to provide.

Target Markets and Entry Strategies

The marketing plan determines the target markets and *market-entry strategies*. Target markets are those consumers that possess a set of distinguishing characteristics to whom your company wants to sell health and fitness services. These characteristics usually refer to certain demographic factors within a geographic service area. Market-entry strategies are those plans that the company will follow to reach consumers and convince them to buy services.

Market Segmentation

The decision on how to position a company is based on market segmentation. Market segmentation is a process that begins with identifying the

Competitors' Comparative Characteristics

Characteristic	Your Company	Competitor A	Competitor B	Competitor C
Geographic boundaries				
Target markets				
Market segmentation procedures				
Marketing strategies and tactics				
Marketing assumptions				
Marketing mix				
Program/products/services offered				
Operating costs/assumptions				
Market share				
Market place entry/exit; stage of life cycle				

Competitor Information Source Outline

I. Competitor Sources

   A. Direct Inquiry

   B. Observation/Facility Visits

   C. Current or Former Employees

   D. Speeches

   E. Company Publications

   F. Press Releases/News Stories

   G. Financial Reports

   H. Investor/Stock Information

   I. Advertisements

   J. Help-Wanted Ads

II. Trade Sources

   A. Trade Organizations

   B. Trade Publications

   C. Trade Shows and Exhibits

   D. Professional Organizations and Meetings

III. Published Sources

   A. Bibliographic Reference Works

   B. Directories

   C. Electronic Data Bases

   D. General Reference Works

   E. Periodicals

   F. University Sources

IV. Third Party Information Sources

   A. Customers

   B. Suppliers

   C. Distributors

   D. Other Competitors

   E. Journalists

   F. Accountants, Consultants, Lawyers

   G. Unions

   H. Your Employees

   I. Security Analysts

   J. Other Sources

target market. That then further specifies the distinguishing characteristics of that chosen market. This will also lead to developing *marketing strategies* and *marketing tactics* that are directed at those customers who seem to be the best potential purchasers of your services. Also, all other aspects of the marketing plan are made more effective by using an appropriate segmentation procedure.

Primary Market Characteristics

Use the following primary characteristics (and those in chapter 2) to segment the market.

Size.   The size of the potential market that will be serviced can be based on either the total volume of dollar sales or the number of possible customers. If this definition of size is not delimiting enough, then the market segment can be broken down further by considering a particular geographic location for the service thrust.

Sociopsychological Needs.   It is often desirable to develop and sell a program or service according to the emotional aspects or needs of the consumer. Every company should be able to identify a consumer desire that can be satisfied from the purchase of one or more programs or services.

Purchaser/User Characteristics.   You must identify the characteristics of both the purchaser and the user. They may not be the same person as would be the case if a company's management contracted with you to provide exercise classes for its employees. A successful provider must become familiar with the characteristics of the purchaser and user, what they both need and want, and how to best satisfy each.

Purchaser Influences.   These are the people, places, and things that will influence consumers in their decision to purchase your services. These influences must be identified, attended to, and satisfied before the consumer will make a purchase.

Service Usage.   It is unfortunate that a health and fitness company must decide to whom they will sell their services on the basis of whether the client can use the services only at the times the company provides them. An important step in segmenting a market according to usage capabilities is to determine whether the clients can use the services when they are offered or whether special provisions must be made. Convenience and flexibility are almost as important to a purchaser's decision to buy as price is.

Buyer Behavior.   Health and fitness services are purchased either on impulse, as when a person joins a local health club or buys a piece of home gym equipment, or with much analysis and planning, as when a company decides to purchase health promotion programs. People buy programs and services to fulfill a variety of needs and for a variety of reasons. Cost will probably be an important factor in all buying decisions as will the method of payment for the purchase. Also, consumer decisions to buy services are based on available (disposable) income.

It would be ideal if market segmentation could occur simply by separating potential targets according to one of these characteristics, but this is not the case. In the health and fitness industry (as well as in most other industries), these components are never separate but rather exist in a combination such as market size and buyer behavior, demographics and geographic location, or purchaser/user characteristics and purchaser influences and usage patterns. The interrelationships among them become more evident and complex as the market segmentation procedure is analyzed in more depth.

Secondary Market Characteristics

Some secondary characteristics that your company may want to use to segment its markets include competition, where the market segment is small but still lacks competition; potential growth, where the segments are expanding at a quick rate; value, where the customers will pay a premium price for the products and services you are offering to make entering the market worthwhile; customer acceptability, which means that your programs and services will be welcomed and accepted by the consumers; ease of market entry, which refers to the company's ability and that of competitors to enter a given market segment; and the number of existing competitors, which determines if the market segment can support another provider (Reibstein, 1985). These secondary factors of market segmentation, when combined with the primary ones, make determining a target market correctly more complex. Fortunately, they also add to the accuracy of properly positioning the company in the chosen market.

Market Positioning Techniques

Companies may position themselves according to the attributes and benefits of their programs and services (cf. Ries & Trout, 1986). Another method of *market positioning* involves the price and quality of programs or services. The price usually will reflect the quality. A third way to position a company is to find a new use for an old service. You do not need to "reinvent the wheel" but only to devise a new way to use it. For example, hospitals that have just entered the health and fitness business probably began by revising their patient and nursing education programs so the programs could be offered as community education (health promotion). Depending on what else was available to the consumer in the hospital's service area, they may have carved out a very profitable niche with this positioning technique.

Other methods of positioning include targeting a specific user group, comparing one company's services to another's, or using a combination of these methods (Reibstein, 1985; Reis & Trout, 1986). The purpose of market positioning is to create a perception in the minds of consumers that your company is the market leader and the consumers must purchase your services to satisfy their needs.

The Marketing Mix

The purpose of the *marketing mix* is to combine several integral elements to achieve a greater market share, a strong competitive position, and a positive image with the target market. The marketing mix consists of the "four Ps" of marketing.

Product (or service)-This is the health and fitness product, program, or service such as health promotion or exercise classes that the consumer wishes to purchase for an agreed-on price because it will satisfy certain needs.

Price-This is the value of the service to the consumer and the cost that will be paid to have the service delivered.

Place-This is the delivery or distribution channel through which the service is provided to the client. The place can be the client's offices, your own facility, a community center, a hotel meeting room, or any other facility that will adequately serve the purpose.

Promotion-This is the series of communications that inform consumers of the existence of the services and their need-satisfying capabilities. The communications include advertising, publicity, public relations, personal sales, and sales promotions.

The four Ps are completely synergistic; that is, the total effect of a good mix is greater than the sum of its parts (Assael, 1985; Murphy & Enis, 1985; Reibstein, 1985). No component can ever stand alone, but each must be developed in conjunction with the others if the marketing mix is to lead to successful marketing strategies and tactics.

Notice how everything in the marketing mix focuses on consumers and on satisfying their needs. This relates directly back to the definition of marketing, which says that an exchange of goods or services is required in which both parties benefit. Thus you can always check the development of your marketing mix by making sure it supports the definition of marketing. The following example will help you better understand the marketing mix process. The target market includes all local corporations with 25 to 50 employees and with no fitness facilities of their own. The product is the service of providing an exercise class (or any type of health and fitness program) twice a week on-site at the corporations' headquarters.

Next, the price of the service must be determined. The first step here is to be aware of what your competitors are doing and then to price accordingly. It is a good idea to price the service equal with or slightly higher than any of the competitors. People will then perceive the new service as a good value. With respect to the exercise class, you must determine whether individuals or the companies will pay and whether payment will be on a per class basis or in whole with one flat rate for the entire program. The payment methods and terms must always be specified with the price. Clients can pay in part or in full; with cash, check, or credit; or by a trade-off of services. Also, a decision must be made about when the clients will have to pay for the services. They can pay at the time the services are provided or within 30 days. These are only some of the possibilities you must consider with regard to pricing your services.

Once you determine these factors you must specify a place where the activity will be conducted. The provider may own a fitness center or an exercise studio or may have to contract with an outside facility. In this example, classes will be offered on-site for the client companies. Determining where the service will be provided is essential because it is the only way the product can be delivered to the client.

Finally, you must consider promotion. Promotion will be discussed in depth in the next chapter, but for now, realize you must identify the advertising, *publicity*, and sales techniques that will inform the potential clients of the service and specify the methods by which new clients will be contacted and contracted and through which current clients will be maintained.

This example gives a brief overview of the proper development of a marketing mix and an associated marketing strategy for providing a corporate exercise program. The techniques are applicable to any health and fitness service situation. Use the marketing mix to develop the marketing strategies and tactics of the marketing plan.

Marketing Strategies and Tactics

The strategies and tactics that will be used in health and fitness *service marketing* were first identified in the strategic analysis section of the business plan, and they should be repeated in this section of your marketing plan. You now have more information to develop the strategies and tactics further. All the data collection that you have completed to this point provides you with the material you need to refine your strategies and tactics for entering and penetrating the market, gaining a competitive advantage, attaining market share, achieving market growth, and making projections for future revenue generation and profitability as the business progresses through the stages of its life cycle. The relationship among these strategic concepts and their recommended tactical areas of implementation is shown in Figure 4.1.

There are many excellent sources of information about marketing strategy and implementation. I have listed a few of the best in the suggested reading list at the end of this book.

This concludes the discussion of the marketing plan components. In chapter 5 promotion and the promotional mix are discussed in detail. The formulation of the correct promotional mix is one of the most important reasons to gather complete marketing information.

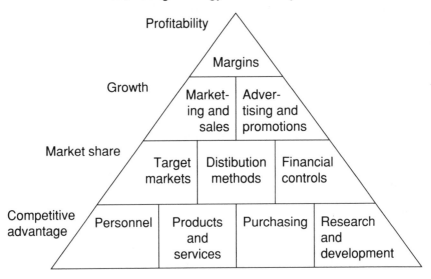

Figure 4.1 Marketing Strategy/Success Pyramid: Strategic concepts and recommended tactical areas of implementation.

Chapter 5

The Promotional Mix

Developing the right promotional mix is critical to any successful marketing plan. How you decide to promote your company's services will be affected by multiple variables—the marketplace, competition, and your company's internal structure. This chapter covers each major type of promotion and the decision-making process for choosing the proper mix of promotional techniques. Two abbreviated marketing plans are presented to demonstrate how each component of the marketing plan, including promotional mix, can be used to develop practical marketing strategies.

Before we examine the promotional mix, basic communication concepts will be discussed. Promotion, after all, depends on communication. Understanding communication fundamentals will help you evaluate your promotional options.

The Communication Process and Promotion

The effectiveness of the entire marketing program, and especially the promotional campaign, depends on the communication process. Everything that is done in marketing is a form of communication—an attempt by the provider to inform the consumer about goods, products, and services. It is essential for health and fitness professionals to be aware of the many steps involved during a communication effort.

The communication process is shown in Figure 5.1, and is based on the 5 Ms: Marketer as source, Message as information, Medium as transmittal channel, Market as consumer audience, and Measurement as feedback (cf., Murphy & Enis, 1985).

The Communication Process

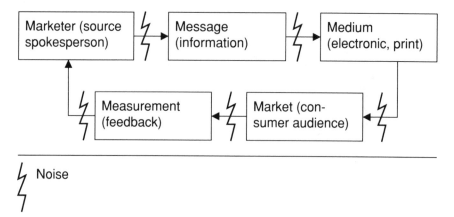

Figure 5.1.   The communication process is based on the five Ms: marketer, message, medium, market, and measurement.

Communication begins when a sender attempts to send a message to a potential customer. The message must be sent in such a way so that the receiver understands and interprets the message in exactly the way it was meant. Because there are several steps in the process between the sender and receiver there are many chances for the process to break down. Usually, noise will deteriorate any message that is sent, so health and fitness marketers must make every effort to eliminate noise in the communication system.

The message that is sent must be encoded, or packaged, in a form that will be easy for the receiver to understand. The message is transmitted through a channel, probably voice, electronic, or print, and then it is decoded by the receiver. You will know that the communication process has successfully been completed when the customer provides feedback that is identical to the message you originally sent.

There are many obstacles that must be overcome when marketing health and fitness services to customers through communication channels. Some of the barriers to effective communication include perceptual distortions between the source and the receiver, a difference in values and attitudes between the people in the communication process, the incorrect use of words or use of improper words to convey specific meanings, and the receiver just not listening to what you are saying. All of these will lead to an improper interpretation of the message you are sending.

In order to ensure effective communication and to be certain that your marketing and advertising message is properly reaching the consumer, you must learn to send messages that are clear and understandable, be aware of potential roadblocks to communication such as noise in the communication system, and listen carefully to the feedback you receive. This last point may be the most important since it requires you to stay in constant contact with your customers. You must also always be aware of their needs, their wants, and what they are telling you. In short, you must be responsive to your customers if you want your marketing and promotional communications to be effective.

The Components of the Promotional Mix

The *promotional mix* activates the strategies and tactics of the marketing plan through five basic components: advertising, *sales promotions*, personal selling, publicity, and public relations. Advertising refers to paid *media* methods that a company uses to inform the buying public that services and programs are available for purchase. Sales promotions include a variety of techniques that introduce consumers to a service and motivate them to buy, usually at a discounted rate. Personal *sales* involve direct contact between a company representative and a potential client. A company owner's or program director's personal sales approach reflects his or her personality, philosophy, and marketing style. Company sales representatives try to match and develop this approach so they can represent the company effectively. Because so much depends on developing an effective personal sales approach, the steps to a personal sale and how to apply them will be examined separately in chapter 6. Publicity refers to free media placements of information on the company, its programs and services, and even its personnel.

The promotional mix combines these five elements to create awareness of the programs and services, to induce clients to try them, and to influence these clients to repurchase the services (Assael, 1985). The success of the mix is totally dependent on the service being offered, its stage in the life cycle, the readiness of the consumer to buy the service, and the methods of communication (paid or unpaid) used to inform the consumers of the availability of the service (Assael, 1985; Bennett, 1988; Kotler, 1988; Reibstein, 1985).

Advertising

Advertising is defined as any paid form of presentation of a company's ideas, products, or services in an impersonal way (Assael, 1985; Kotler,

1988; Murphy & Enis, 1985). It is impersonal because there is no person-to-person contact. Advertising is done through newspapers, radio, television, magazines, direct mail, brochures, fliers, forms, displays, and *word of mouth*. These methods present your company's message, but there is no way actually to measure their impact because you cannot always determine whether a client purchased a program or service as a result of the advertising campaign or of some other influence. Of course, most people assume that increased sales should be due to the advertising effort, but this is not always the case. Increased sales can often be the result of other promotional techniques or simply of personal referrals. Whatever the case, your company must try to fulfill one or several objectives with its advertising campaign.

The first objective is to publicize the program or service. The goal is to inform the consumers of your service and to show how it can satisfy their needs. This objective can be met by advertising either one program or service or an entire product line. For example, there are several companies that try to influence clients to purchase their entire line of health promotion programs such as weight control, stress management, and smoking cessation, whereas other companies advertise only one of these programs. Each is trying to fulfill this first objective of informing the buying public of the availability of health promotion programs and their need-satisfying capabilities.

The second objective of an advertising campaign is to increase the demand for a program or service to cause an increase in sales, a possible increase in prices, or a transfer of customer loyalty from competitors to your company (Bennett, 1988; Kotler, 1988; Reibstein, 1985). If this objective is met, then the third objective of advertising would directly follow: to create a recognizable name and a positive image of the company. Because this is also an objective of public relations, the advertising and public relations efforts will support each other.

There are other objectives that an advertising program may try to achieve. Public information and employee motivation are two examples. These objectives will be achieved differently depending on whether a product or service is being advertised. Therefore, health and fitness providers must understand the difference between product advertising and service advertising.

Product and Service Advertising

Product advertising is actually quite simple. A company has a tangible product that it wishes to inform the public about; the company develops ads to communicate this information and even shows a picture of the product in the ad. You can see product advertising in any trade journal in the health and fitness profession. There are ads for bicycles, treadmills, weights, health promotion programs with workbooks and leaders' guides, and many other tangible items.

Service advertising is more difficult because ads cannot show the service in action. Services are intangible, variable, and they are consumed at the time of purchase. They cannot be stored for later use. This makes it difficult to identify the differences among companies in the same profession. Marcus (1986) has recommended that service companies follow some basic advertising rules:

- Develop the ad in terms of the clients' needs, not of the company that places it.
- Address only one service in each ad.
- Keep the ads local even if the company is national.
- Define the service as if the company were the first to offer it.
- Place the ads on a regular basis.
- Be honest and open in describing the services and programs that the company is offering.

The health and fitness companies that follows these rules will achieve a measurable level of success. However, most companies do not have the in-house capabilities to generate professional, attention-getting ads. They must hire an outside advertising agency. Weinrauch (1987) suggests that to determine which agency best fits your company's needs you should identify the skills of the agency's personnel; their understanding of your programs and services and how you are trying to promote them; their ability to provide all the services that your company may need, such as ad production, copywriting, placements, market research, and creative work; their past success with similar companies in the health and fitness field; any conflicts of interest with the agency's other accounts; their ability to meet deadlines; their procedure for tracking the results and impact of the advertising campaign; their methods for charging and billing for their work; their payment terms; and their techniques for reporting information to you. Then you must interview the agency and be satisfied that their representatives interact well with your staff.

Media Selection

Media selection determines the method through which information about your company is communicated to the public. The most common media are television, radio, newspapers, magazines, brochures, fliers, billboards, direct mail, telemarketing, and word of mouth. Most companies think in terms of placing their ads in the three main media: television, radio, and print (usually newspapers or magazines).

While these three methods are those most commonly used, the power of word-of-mouth advertising should never be underestimated. This is especially true for companies that rely on memberships for most of their revenue. Media advertising is helpful in informing the public that the facility exists and that memberships are available, but club owners know that most of their new members will come from referrals from current members (IRSA, 1985). Whichever media format is chosen, it should be selected according to six criteria (Reibstein, 1985):

Selectivity. This refers to the medium's ability to reach a specific geographic segment or target market. If your company wants to provide health promotion programs to hospitals, you may consider placing an ad in a special health care section of the local newspaper. This section is usually targeted for hospitals and other health care consumers and providers.

Penetration. This is the extent to which the medium actually reaches the target market. You can determine the effectiveness of the placements by tracking the responses to the advertisement.

Coverage. This is the percentage of the total market that a medium is able to reach. If your ad is placed in a regional issue of the newspaper, it should reach 100% of the readership in that area.

Flexibility. The flexibility of a medium is determined by how far in advance an advertising commitment must be made. Newspapers and radio are usually more flexible than television is.

Cost. This is usually the most important determinant of which medium to choose. There are times when the cost of using a particular medium is prohibitive, such as television during the Super Bowl. You must therefore select a less expensive medium yet one that meets the other criteria in accordance with the marketing objectives of the company. Most health and fitness companies tend to purchase print space, which often is the most cost-effective. But you may want to consider the cost of using smaller print ads and supplementing them with radio advertisements.

Editorial Environment. This determines the tone or the setting in which the advertisement appears and thus how it is perceived by the target audience. Media with both high audience acceptance and high perceived credibility should always be considered. Consumers will associate their positive perceptions of a particular medium with the programs or services that are advertised in it. If you place an ad in *The Wall Street Journal* or *The New York Times* to inform executives of your health and fitness programs you will get a better response and be perceived as more credible than if your ad were placed in one of the supermarket tabloids.

Maintaining a Realistic Approach

A health and fitness company should never enter an advertising campaign with lofty ideals of what will be accomplished. There are certain things that advertising can and cannot do for a company (Marcus, 1986; Weinrauch, 1987). Advertising can give the company the opportunity to say what it wants. (This lacks full credibility, however, because the consumer knows that the ad space and time were purchased.) Advertising can inform the public about a company's programs and services and can help create name recognition, a positive image, and reputation for the company. It can also generate some kind of action by the consumer through its persuasive messages. But advertising cannot work without an overall marketing plan, nor can it close a sale due to its impersonal nature. Ten advertising techniques to help you develop more effective campaigns follow.

- Position the program or service so the consumer identifies it with a name or slogan. For example, "Freedom from Smoking" is identified with the American Lung Association.
- The advertising budget should be designed according to how much revenue is needed to reach a specific sales objective. Using percentage of sales to determine your advertising budget is not recommended because advertising is supposed to produce sales, not vice versa. You must determine through research, trial and success, and sometimes plain luck the costs of informing the public of your products and services so that a certain amount of revenue will be generated.
- There are times when you should present competitors' ads to consumers before yours. This can be done by either the advertising agency or your staff. Simply ask people what they think about a particular ad. Get them to discuss what they like or dislike about it. Their opinions will identify the strengths and weaknesses of the products or services they are being asked to purchase. You can then create more appropriate ads on the basis of this information.
- The headline of an ad is very important. Begin the headline with "Which . . ." It is difficult to write a bad headline or ad when it begins with "Which." Suppose you wanted to sell a weight control program and your ad's headline read, "Do you want to lose weight?" If the reader has no interest in losing weight, he or she will read no further and you will have lost a potential customer. Now change the headline to read, "Which method of losing weight do you prefer?" You have now captured the attention of readers who want to lose weight and even some of those who previously had no desire to do so.
- The headline must contain information that you want to convey to

consumers (such as helping them lose weight). The rest of the ad must be written so that it is closely tied to the headline. Once someone has become interested in a headline, they often will take the time to read the entire ad, especially if they feel that the ad addresses them personally.

- Write ads so that they are directed toward prime customers. Close every ad with a phrase or slogan that will be remembered. Many companies close their ads with the phrase "Adding quality to your years," which tells customers that, although the programs may not extend their lives, they will make their lives more enjoyable.

- Keep print-ad sizes down and supplement them with radio spots. This will expand your audience. You must, however, make this decision on the basis of your marketing objectives and budget.

- Tell people what they want to hear but do not make any claims about programs or services that cannot be supported. People want to hear that they can lose weight, control their stress levels, get in shape, and stop smoking. Tell them how you can help them achieve those goals but be honest, sincere, and professional and provide support for your statements.

- Be ready to alter ads as the audience or media tools change. For example, newspaper ads may have been successful, but now you need to modify your approach because you do not seem to be reaching your audience. One suggestion is to go to a direct-mail piece—a letter or a brochure—that is sent to the homes of potential clients. This ensures their receiving your information and becoming aware of your services.

- Evaluate your advertising program periodically and make adjustments where necessary. Advertising is a campaign, or a series of ads, not just a one-shot deal. The ads must change as the audience or your message changes. For example, consider a health and fitness center that is located in the north. Its ads have been bringing in memberships through the fall and spring, but, for some reason, people have not been joining in the winter and summer, perhaps because it is too cold to go out in the winter and they prefer to enjoy the outdoors in the summer. One service the facility can offer is to have its staff work as personal trainers who go to people's homes in the winter and lead them through an exercise program or who will serve as group leaders for outdoor exercise programs in the summer. This is one of many options for altering an advertising campaign. It also provides an alternative revenue source.

No matter how you choose to advertise or which agency you choose to work with, the advertising campaign will be based on the "four Ms" of advertising:

Media: The method you will use to get your message across

Message: The information you are trying to convey

Market: The people you are trying to reach with the message

Money: The actual cost of the advertising campaign

Advertising programs must be supported by a variety of other promotional techniques, including sales promotions, publicity, and public relations. Each of these will be discussed in relation to the marketing plan in general and the promotional mix in particular.

Before reading about each area of promotion, study this list of image-building ideas and see how many more you can imagine. They all can be considered a form of advertising. Also consider all the steps needed to implement these ideas.

- Newspapers: articles, editorials, quotations, display and classified advertising
- Magazines: consumer, trade, association, and local and society publications including ads and stories about the company
- Telephone directories: Yellow Pages and specialty directories
- Direct mail: letters, cards, leaflets, brochures, and catalogs
- Radio and television: live and prerecorded messages and commercials
- Outdoor advertising: billboards, posters, signs, and handbills
- Specialty items: calendars, pens, pencils, cups, key chains, and other premium, or "remembrance," items
- Exhibits and trade shows: regional and national trade shows, local civic exhibits, and other types of public displays
- Speeches: company representatives speaking to civic, business, and professional organizations
- *Networking*: meeting anyone who has skills, contacts, or connections that can be advantageous to you and to whom you can provide the same benefit

Keep in mind that the result of a good marketing and advertising campaign is a confirmed sale. Methods to actually "make the sale" of your programs and services will be discussed in the next chapter.

Sales Promotions

Promotions are nonpersonal communications that supplement and complement advertising and personal selling (Kotler, 1988; Weinrauch, 1987), thus making them more effective. Promotions are similar to advertising in that they attempt to communicate information to potential customers about the need-satisfying capabilities of a program or service. Promotions are not paid-for placements in a medium but often are company-sponsored programs that are designed to influence consumers to purchase by offering an incentive. Many of the incentives in the health and fitness industry involve sales-related items such as program or club membership discounts, rebates, coupons, premiums (gifts or prizes with the purchase of a program or service), and even free or short-term trial memberships. The incentive to participate in a promotional event is that clients will receive either a financial or a personal gain as a result of their involvement.

Any sales promotion campaign has several objectives. These include stimulating immediate sales, creating a sense of consumer urgency to purchase the service, encouraging consumers to buy more of the service than they would normally have bought, and producing temporary excitement in the market (Weinrauch, 1987). The effective use of sales promotions is limited by the constraints of the overall marketing plan and by the budgetary guidelines established for promotion. The following example should help clarify how to meet promotional objectives.

You have only several hundred dollars to spend for a sales promotion of a new weight-loss program you want to offer, and you obviously need to inform the public about it. First, you can place a newspaper ad that announces the program and a free lecture that will be given to describe it. You can also include a discount coupon for the program to get people to attend the lecture and sign up. Second, you can place a public service announcement in the newspaper's calendar of events. This placement is free because you are informing the public about an activity in the community. Third, you can spend some of the money on T-shirts that carry the name and logo of the weight-loss program and have employees and others wear the shirts whenever possible. Finally, you can have radio and television stations mention the free lecture, and then you can use the lecture as your promotional tool to sell the program. This should not cost anything because it is a public service announcement for a free service.

Sales promotions of this type as well as other ones can be very beneficial to your company. However, it is important for all health and fitness companies to remember that they must not oversaturate the market with constant sales promotions. Promotions must be used strategically, or they will not increase consumer demand for the services. Ongoing promotions may be perceived by consumers as a ploy to get them to purchase an inferior product. Strategically placed promotions will convince consumers (both new and repeat) to buy the program or service, if only to try it out. This is especially true if the promotion is a discount or a guaranteed refund. People tend to buy more of a product or to try a new product if there is little or no financial risk involved.

Companies should also remember that carefully designed and timed promotions can stimulate short-term sales when there is actually little demand for the services. For example, it is a well-known fact that club usage and memberships drop off during the summer. Many clubs therefore promote special summertime memberships such as use of the facility for a dollar a day, reduced rates for students, or a free summer's use of the club for purchasing a 1-year membership. The same approach can be followed by every company in the health and fitness industry regardless of the service being offered. Just be sure that the sales promotions match the company's marketing and advertising objectives.

Publicity

Many of the methods of promoting your programs and services involve publicity. Publicity is a form of communication designed to influence consumer buying behavior, like advertising, but it is neither sponsored by the company nor necessarily designed to stimulate sales (Bennett, 1988; Kotler, 1988; Reibstein, 1985). Theoretically, it is free. Publicity involves media exposure for the company that is basically nonsponsored and unpaid-for ''advertising.'' The main goal of any publicity campaign is to increase the name recognition and credibility of the company and, combined with public relations, to create a favorable and positive image.

There are many ways that a company can receive publicity. The staff may be viewed as a reliable resource for information in the health and fitness field. Then newspaper, television, and radio reporters might seek out company representatives to help them with a story. Or the company may be viewed as the authoritative source on a subject and as having so much credibility that the media chooses to produce a story about them. The company may also be offering a new type of service or an old service with a new twist that a broadcast medium may think is newsworthy. Also, companies may send news releases to inform the press about major events or may even hold press conferences to do the same. Whatever method is chosen, the idea remains the same, that is, to get someone else to tell the consumer about your company without you having to pay for it.

All of this may sound simple, but it can actually be very difficult. Newspapers and radio and television stations would rather fill their advertising space with paid advertising than free publicity. Therefore, the company must appoint someone to carry out the publicity function and convince the media of the value of what you are offering. This person must feel comfortable with contacting every possible source of free publicity. But remember that publicity will be forthcoming only if it pertains to worthwhile information. The following example shows a way for a health and fitness company to gain publicity.

A hospital-based health and fitness center was contacted by a local newspaper to advertise in its special executive health care section. This section was targeted to a market that the center was trying to reach, and advertising dollars had been allocated for the ad's placement. The newspaper already considered the center a credible resource, and the center decided to support its advertising by having staff members write articles for the newspaper's health care section as well as serve as resources for the newspaper's reporters. The editors of the newspaper thought this was a good idea, a way that both parties could benefit. The center received five other free publicity placements (articles about the center that mention it as an expert resource) in addition to the paid advertising.

You must think of publicity as an integral part of the overall marketing program, and it must be used strategically. If your company thinks that everything it does is worth free publicity, and it informs the media accordingly, the media might begin to view your company as self-serving. Then, when you have something truly newsworthy to offer to consumers, the media may not provide the publicity for fear it is simply another unwarranted request. So plan the publicity campaign carefully, use the various methods judiciously, maintain the company's position as a credible resource of information on health and fitness, and always use positive public relations to augment your publicity campaign.

Public Relations

The primary goal of public relations is to foster a positive image of the company in the minds of consumers. This definition seems simple, yet public relations is perhaps the most misunderstood concept in the entire promotional mix. Public relations is often confused with advertising, which it definitely is not, and with publicity, which it may result in or may lead to. Public relations involves forms of communication that cost your company in a different way than do advertising or sales promotions. You need to consider costs such as personnel salaries, planning time, program development, and program implementation as well as office supplies, telephone, travel, and other business-related expenses. Many of these are intangible expenses and are often forgotten in the marketing plan's budget. You must make money available for public relations in the same way that money is allocated for advertising and sales promotions.

Because many companies in the health and fitness industry offer similar programs and services, it is important to differentiate your public relations effort by informing consumers of the high-quality programs and services you are offering. Focus on client contact and service before, during, and after the sale, especially as repeat business often is a function of follow-up service (Peters, 1987). A successful public relations program will be based on the following criteria (Marcus, 1986):

- It exposes and projects the company's greatest strengths and capabilities to the community and in particular to the target market.
- It emphasizes the company's expertise in the health and fitness industry as well as the quality of its service.
- It competes successfully with the public relations efforts of competitors.
- It allows for the measurement and evaluation of the information it provides to the target markets.
- It is done in-house, or, if an outside agency is used, the program still remains internally driven.

Health and fitness companies should begin their public relations programs using internal resources due to the high cost of contracting with an outside professional agency. The following example explains a public relations campaign that was used to enhance a company's image and reputation.

A health and fitness provider wanted to provide local businesses with employee exercise programs. The standard method of contacting a client is by either telephone or direct mail, but both of these can be costly. Instead, the provider volunteered its staff to perform an exercise demonstration in conjunction with a local, well-known charity. The charity and the exercise demonstration were scheduled to receive media coverage. Also, the provider contacted several current and prospective clients and invited them to the demonstration. This gave everyone who attended a positive image of the company as charitable, community minded, and service oriented. Furthermore, many other people were expected to attend the charity event and would see the exercise demonstration, and would be potential clients. This would plant the idea for employee exercise programs in their minds and they could be contacted to determine further interest. Finally, the follow-up publicity and news coverage of the event further enhanced the image, reputation, and credibility of the company, thereby making the public relations effort worthwhile.

This example typifies a successful public relations campaign. One other type of public relations/publicity technique that must be discussed is *networking*. This is perhaps one of the most effective yet least used methods. Networking involves people meeting people and talking about and to each other. These people usually have skills or contacts that can benefit you, and you can do the same for them. So meet as many people as possible. Go to business, community, Chamber of Commerce, and social meetings. Give everyone you meet a business card, which is the second-least expensive form of advertising and public relations yet is often underutilized. Make sure that the business card expresses the company's message adequately and introduces the person who carries it. Never underestimate the power of networking or word-of-mouth advertising, which can lead you to potential clients at the most unlikely times. Be seen and be heard and let others do your selling for you whenever possible.

The value of a good promotional program in general and of a good public relations campaign in particular is seen in the results. Program effectiveness is determined by heightened consumer awareness about your company's services, increased sales, reduced selling costs due to an increased volume of business, establishment of the company as the primary resource for health and fitness information and services, enhanced community good will, a respected and credible reputation, increased consumer inquiries and prospective buyers for the services, and the development of an expanded client list.

These results can also be achieved through informal public relations simply by having your staff be very personable to everyone they meet. The personal touch, which is commonly lacking in advertising and sales promotions, will greatly improve the formal public relations campaign and lend support to the advertising program. The costs of all these efforts must always be considered. See the advertising cost plan form for a suggested month-by-month expense format. List all the promotional avenues you might use during a given month and record the amount you spend each month throughout the year.

Finally, everything a company does should be considered public relations. Contacts with current clients, the provision of programs and services, publicity, and so on are the more obvious and perhaps more tangible methods of public relations. But less obvious techniques may become powerful buyer influences, including office decor, stationery, staff dress, manners of speech, and body language. If there is uncertainty about how to deal with these influences, just remember to keep everything professional, positive, upbeat, and friendly, and the desired results will come naturally.

A Sample Facility Marketing Plan

I have included two abbreviated sample marketing plans* here so you will be able to see how the guidelines presented in chapters 4 and 5 relate to actual marketing situations. The first plan is for a facility-based company. This plan shows how a small health and fitness center can inform the public of its services and increase its revenues and profits. I would like you to note that while this plan is written according to the guidelines of this book, it differs in some areas from the strict presentation found in the text. This is as it should be, for every business and every market differs according to its specific strengths, weaknesses, market place, and position within the industry.

---

*Because both of these plans are designed to represent only the organizational and writing processes, support documentation has not been included.

Advertising Cost Plan 19___

Media	Dollar amount by month											
	Jan	Feb	Mar	Apr	May	Jun	Jul	Aug	Sep	Oct	Nov	Dec
Newspaper												
Radio												
Television												
Magazine												
Direct mail												
Brochures/flyers												
Other												

Executive Summary

The health and fitness facility is located in a small town in the Southeast. It is the only facility in the town and caters to approximately 10,000 residents in a five-square-mile radius. The club has 500 annual members who pay a yearly fee of $250. The company has been in operation for 4 years. It has had no formal marketing program in any of these years. Its main advertising consists of a roadside sign in front of the facility that reads "Fitness" in 6-inch-high letters and single-page 3″ x 8″ brochures that include a list of its programs and services.

The major goals of the marketing plan are to (a) help the club become more profitable by increasing its membership base, (b) increase the number of guests who use the facility while visiting the town, (c) develop new and innovative programs such as health promotion and senior exercise classes, and (d) expand the club's services beyond the current geographic boundaries. All this must be accomplished with an annual marketing budget of $7,500.

The potential is good for significant profits for the club. It has a strong competitive position as it is the only fitness center in the town. The nearest competition is almost 10 miles away in another city. One goal of the marketing plan is to provide methods to attract this competitor's members to the club to join as members. This will also help it reach another goal: to achieve a 10% market share (1,000 members) within the calendar year.

Market Segmentation Procedures

The market segmentation procedures used by the club are relatively simple. The club accepts members on the basis of age, income, education, type of lifestyle, and facility accessibility. The people who live in the area can definitely afford the membership fees. Therefore, market segmentation need not be done in an overly scientific way.

Market Analysis

This portion of the plan will describe the company's market research, assessment of demand, and analysis of the industry life cycle.

Market Research

The club has never conducted formal market research programs. Its only methods of data collection prior to the current year were personal discussions with members, town residents, and guests and a request for these people to fill out a brief questionnaire at the club.

The club will engage in one small market research program near the end of the current year in the form of a short survey to be sent to annual members and guests about the programs and services offered by the club and the price structure of membership dues. This survey will be written and formalized so that the responses can be analyzed statistically. The goal of this survey is to provide the staff with enough information about the types of programs in which people want to participate, what they are willing to pay for those programs, and how much the annual membership dues can be raised prior to the start of the next year.

Market Demand

The club caters to young professionals who have already made fitness a major part of their lives and to some active retirees. The club also caters to guests who maintain a fitness program at home or who want to begin one while on vacation.

The club needs to open other markets to continue to be successful. These include the corporate market, the women's market, and currently inactive seniors.

Industry Life Cycle

The status of the fitness industry is the same for all clubs. The industry is still in the early growth stages of its development as evidenced by the increasing numbers of people who are beginning exercise programs, maintaining their current ones, and venturing into new training areas such as cross-training for triathlons.

These life-cycle indicators show the tremendous market demand for fitness services. It is imperative that the club be responsive to these demands by upgrading the quality of its current programs and services and by instituting new ones as well. Currently, the club is in a strong competitive position and finds its market very attractive. But changes can occur rapidly, and the club must be able to enter new markets and expand its current ones. The approach that the club will take to control its market share is one of innovation and quality service so that it can easily enter new markets, penetrate more deeply in new and current ones, and easily exit from any that are not profitable.

Company Analysis

This is a relatively small company with only two full-time employees: a club manager and a front-desk receptionist. There are usually between 5 and 10 part-time employees, depending on the need. The club is able to service its annual members during slow periods with no more than five part-time staff members who are cross-trained to work in every area of the facility.

The club describes itself as a comprehensive health/fitness facility with weight-training and cardiovascular equipment, aerobics classes, suntanning room, lockers, and shower rooms. The facility is about 5,000 square feet. Its stated comprehensiveness is related more to the activities and services it provides than to its size. The club is further defined by its management philosophy and staff-client interactions. Management believes in being directly involved with the daily activities, and the club manager works the exercise floor and teaches aerobics classes. The staff is friendly, well trained, and genuinely interested in working with the clients. No member works out alone or is unsupervised. A unique feature of the club (and this is probably due to its small size and small membership base) is that every staff member knows every annual member by name. Management trusts and supports the staff, who, in return, support the clients and provides for them well.

The club, like any health club, has its limitations and weaknesses. Management feels that it could provide more services if the facility, especially the locker-room areas, were larger. It also would like a larger sign on the main road, but the decision to install one is controlled by a city ordinance and by the owner of the plaza in which the club leases its space.

Another weakness that the club's management is trying to correct is its inability to attract quality aerobics instructors. Many instructors do not want to teach in small facilities and opt for larger clubs with more people per class. Another related problem is that the club manager has high standards of performance for aerobics instructors, and many instructors at other clubs do not meet those standards. One solution is to pay certified aerobics instructors $12 to $15 per class and to require that they attend at least one training seminar per month at the club. This will attract the better aerobics instructors and also allow the club to maintain its quality standards of performance and control.

Competitor Analysis

The competitor analysis for the club is relatively simple. There are no other facilities within five square miles that provide such a wide variety of programs and services. The nearest competitor, and probably the primary one, is more than 10 miles away. This fitness center provides programs similar to those offered at the club. The competitor is 4 years old, about 40,000 square feet, and was built at a cost of over $3 million. It contains all the amenities such as whirlpools, plunge pools, saunas, and steam baths. Although the membership of the center is not especially large, it does affect the size of the club simply because people who drive between towns stop at the competitor's facility on their way to or from work. Another membership attraction is that one may buy a tennis membership with a fitness center membership.

The club also has some minor, or secondary, competitors. These competing clubs are located in other cities 15 to 20 miles away. They include a typical health and fitness center and a hospital wellness center. Membership prices and the range of services vary at each of these facilities as do the numbers of members. The club does not consider these facilities to be true competitors simply because they are so far away.

Program and Service Analysis

The club currently offers two types of programs, both of which are based on supervision and personalized service. The first is a strength-training program using Nautilus machines and free weights. The staff is always present to help members use the equipment properly and get the most out of their workouts.

The second program comprises a variety of low-impact aerobics classes that are taught by certified aerobics instructors (who also must complete a training program developed by the club manager). The classes are designed to accommodate all fitness levels and age groups.

Marketing Strategies and Tactics

This portion of the plan will cover marketing objectives, business goals, and marketing strategies and tactics.

Marketing Objectives

The club has simple marketing objectives. It seeks to secure a 10% market share of the town population as members. This will provide them with a base membership of 1,000 people, which will further secure their competitive advantage. This will also allow them to take the initiative in setting membership rates and prices for auxiliary programs.

Business Goals

The business goals for the club are threefold. The first is to achieve a break-even point solely from membership sales by the end of the current year. The second goal is to develop alternative revenue sources by offering health promotion programs and services at local businesses. These revenues will be used to assist the club in making a profit. The third goal is to receive income from educational and training workshops that the club will sponsor throughout the area.

The financial goals of the club are not difficult to achieve. In fact, the club will be satisfied with an operating expense ratio that is 66% of gross revenues. This will ensure them a small but definite after-tax profit of about 10% to 15%. The profits will then be reinvested into the business to upgrade the facility and to expand the external market base by providing more programs and services.

Marketing Strategies

The marketing strategies relate to activities in which the club will engage to maintain service for their clients and to add subsequent program and service offerings that will help maximize the club's position as a health and fitness provider. The primary corporate strategy is to continue selling memberships through minimal external advertising. The plan is to develop an effective membership referral system that will bring more people into the club. The corollary to annual membership sales is short-term or monthly memberships. These provide another source of cash flow for the facility.

Marketing Tactics

The marketing strategies will be implemented through a minimum of print advertising and a maximum of free publicity. Other tactics include upgrading the member referral program, developing special memberships for specific age groups, and providing the best possible service of any of the fitness centers in the area.

The marketing mix that the club will use includes offering facility memberships at $250 per year plus additional fees for specialty programs such as stress management or weight control. Other price schedules for short-term memberships are based on the length of the membership. A unique feature of the club's program offerings is that the staff is capable of providing any or all of the programs at another site. For example, if a corporation requests a daily aerobics class, the club will send one of its instructors to that company at the agreed-on time to teach the class at a predetermined price. This ability to distribute its programs and services off-site is one of the attributes that will make the club the definite market leader by the end of the current year.

The tactics for implementing the marketing strategies are sound. The club will control the marketing plan by doing only a few things at a time so that the effectiveness of its efforts can be evaluated. The club will contact three companies per week to arrange exercise classes and educational lectures for their employees. This is tracked on the basis of whether the club gets the service contract. The membership referral program is controlled by requesting guests or new members to identify the current member who referred them. Of course, these tracking methods must be reflected in increased revenues for the strategies and tactics to be considered effective.

If the control procedure identifies a strategy or tactic that is not effective, that is, not helping the club achieve its marketing or financial goals, then the club will either adapt the weak strategy or tactic or develop a new one as a replacement. The strong competitive position that the club is now in allows it to test its markets continually and to be flexible in whatever it decides to do.

Promotional Mix

The club engages in a limited print advertising and publicity program. It would not be advantageous for the club to purchase ad space in papers outside the town because the cost would be too prohibitive for the return the club would receive. However, the club manager writes a regular fitness column for the town newspaper and always includes the club in the byline. This serves as a form of both advertising and publicity.

Advertising

The only true print advertising that the club conducts is its distribution of brochures, which are given out at the club and at selected retail locations in the town. The club also has a listing on the Chamber of Commerce computer file that serves as an "electronic brochure."

One other type of advertising the club engages in is direct mail to residents and members. This direct-mail piece explains the programs the club is offering as well as special promotions such as discounted memberships for seniors. The club has also begun a direct-mail joint venture with a local hotel operator that places club brochures in all the hotel's sales packets. This mail reaches a previously untapped market because business travelers are always looking for a place to exercise. The club manager will contact other hotels to arrange similar placements in their sales packets.

Publicity

The publicity that the club receives is excellent. The club manager is respected in the community and is looked on by the newspapers, television, and radio media as *the* local fitness expert. The manager is often requested to appear on shows and to serve as a resource for articles on fitness and health.

The club also sends out news releases whenever it begins a new program or service. For example, a news release on their Club 55 senior exercise program will be sent to all the media representatives every year. The goal is to receive as much exposure as possible for the program and to inform seniors that the club is willing to cater to their special needs.

The club also ties much of its publicity efforts to charitable activities. The aerobics instructors volunteer to perform at various functions. The club has also developed cooperative relationships with many of the retailers in the town. The club may provide a trial or a discounted membership for a retailer's employee while the retailer sells goods to club members at reduced prices. This is a win-win situation for everyone. The actions of both the club and the retailer are made known to the local media, and the free publicity supports both businesses.

Public Relations

The club is constantly involved in public relations efforts, especially because the community is relatively small. The staff volunteers for community duties, and the club sponsors community events. This has resulted in a positive public image for the club.

Direct Sales

The club uses only two methods of direct sales, and it plans to maintain this effort because it has proven successful. The first method is to take guests through a tour of the facility. The guests are given all the necessary information about the programs and services and then are provided with membership information. The membership sale is not high pressured. Rather, the philosophy is that the club will sell itself.

The second method of direct sales involves a 3-step approach taken by the club manager. First, the manager sends a letter to a hotel or a major employer in the town that describes the club's services. This is followed up with a telephone call to the client's decision maker to schedule an appointment. Then the manager meets with the client and attempts to sell the programs and services either on-site at the client's location or at the club.

Sales Promotions

Sales promotions efforts are simple yet effective. Therefore, management sees no reason to change them in the coming year. All the staff members leave brochures and discount coupons at retail outlets throughout the community that are for membership price reductions, aerobics class price reductions, or reductions in the fees for health promotion programs. The discounts are never more than 20%, so the club does not lose much when the coupons are redeemed. In fact, the club more than makes up for the discount in the volume of business that is generated.

The club also engages in "typical" club promotions, such as membership referral programs and membership incentive programs. Winning members in each of these programs have received prizes such as aerobics shoes, extensions on membership, and cruises for two.

These promotions have proven successful for the club because they have kept the name of the club visible to all the members and have maintained the club's reputation as one that services its members. One goal for the current year is to expand the sales promotions by getting a retailer or major vendor to cosponsor a membership drive and/or an incentive program. The retailer will be expected to provide the major prize for the winner, such as racing bicycles or a 1-week cruise for two. The club will negotiate this program with several sponsors throughout the year, during which time several promotions will be run if enough sponsors are interested.

Promotional Mix Summary

The parts of the promotional mix include advertising, publicity, public relations, direct sales, and sales promotions. The club has chosen to operate on a budget of $7,500 for the entire calendar year. Although $7,500 may seem insufficient, it is a 50% increase from the previous year's budget. The budget will also be adequate to reach the goals the club wants to achieve with its communication programs.

The budget allocates 20% of the funds for advertising (including brochures and direct-mail pieces), 10% for direct-sales efforts, 60% for sales promotions, and 10% for miscellaneous expenses. The club expects that all publicity and public relations efforts will be free or will come as the result of other activities. Another breakdown of the promotional mix involves effort expenditure. About 50% of all energies will be directed toward gaining additional publicity and furthering the positive image of the club, which, in turn, should lead to an increased membership. The staff will place 25% of their efforts into sales promotions, 15% into direct sales, and 10% into advertising campaigns. Club management has learned from experience that word-of-mouth advertising by their members and by the retailers with whom the club enjoys a positive relationship is the best type of advertising and promotion.

Marketing Results

It is easy to specify the club's membership goal for the current year. The club wants to increase its base from 500 to about 1,000 members. The actual sales revenue that the new memberships will generate is difficult to determine due to the variety of promotions that the club engages in and to the discount programs that are offered. If the club considers $250 per year to be the average membership price, then sales revenue from memberships should be about $250,000.

Obviously, the marketing program will need to generate more sales revenue for the club to sustain a net profit. Additional revenue will be generated when the club enters the corporate market, when health promotion programs for members and employers are provided, and when exercise classes are offered at hotels and corporate sites. This is all uncharted territory for the club as far as programming and income are concerned. Therefore, the sales goal for all these additional revenue sources is a modest $25,000 for the year.

Profits

Management realizes that the club is still in the early stages of its growth. The profit goal for the year is between 5% and 10% of net income. The club also has the capability of realizing more profit through a proliferation of its programs and services to outside clients. The more classes or educational seminars the staff can provide, the greater the profit will be simply because the cost of providing them is fixed. Because there is no history of the club providing these services for clients, it is difficult to determine the actual revenues and profit potential. But management has decided to maintain the goal of a 5% to 10% net profit margin for all its revenue sources. This will give the club a consistent basis from which to track its efforts. It can then modify its goals accordingly.

Differential Advantage

The club enjoys a unique competitive advantage in that it is the only health and fitness center in a five square mile radius. Not only does the club enjoy the largest market share, but it also holds the top competitive position. When the club achieves its membership revenue and profit goals for the year, it may consider expanding to a larger facility.

Recommendations for Future Opportunities

The future of the club looks bright. It is the only fitness facility in the area, and it has an excellent reputation with the members and business community. This alone will bring it more members. Most of the opportunities to increase membership are in special population and corporate memberships.

The club should also try to offer health promotion programs to the major employers in the town, including city and county employees.

Possible expansion includes either enlarging the present facility with more amenities and workout areas or opening another facility in one of several locations. The recommendation is *not* to expand in either of these directions for at least 2 years. The club must first prove that it can implement and profit from the ideas and programs set forth in this marketing plan at its original location before it begins to expand.

The final recommendation for the club is to keep doing what it does well. The club has an excellent reputation for servicing its members, and this should continue. The quality of service of all its programs must be high. Then, when the club is even more firmly established as the area's top provider of health and fitness services, management can consider price increases and expansion. It is expected to take at least 2 years for the club to fully achieve its marketing goals, at which time the plan will need revision.

A Sample Product Marketing Plan

This sample marketing plan is for a fitness equipment manufacturer. The company is SPRI Products, Inc., which produces rubber resistance equipment. Its two primary products include the Xercise Band and Xercise Tubing. The purpose of including this plan is twofold: to demonstrate the differences and similarities of marketing products and marketing facility-based services; and, to show the differences and similarities in creating a marketing plan for a company that is in an early stage of development and creating a plan for one that is in a later stage of development.

Executive Summary

SPRI Products, Inc., is a 4-year-old company that specializes in manufacturing and distributing rubber resistance exercise equipment. The product trade names are Xercise Bands and Xercise Tubing. The company is known primarily for its Xercise Bands, which are used in exercise and rehabilitation programs more than the tubing is. But a major effort is currently under way to introduce the tubing to these training programs.

The primary markets for the products are physical therapists and aerobics instructors, and the products are well accepted by them. The company now wants to expand into the corporate and the hospital-based health and fitness markets.

The rationale for the current marketing plan is that SPRI has never had a formal plan of action by which to communicate the capabilities of its products to consumers. The company relies on trade shows, word of mouth, publicity, trade journal publications, books, and videos to inform the buying public about the bands and tubing. However, several competitors entered the market last year, and, whereas SPRI was once the market leader, it now has to compete for this position with these well-funded businesses. So the company decided that it was necessary to enter new markets to maintain its competitive advantage.

The gross revenue predictions for SPRI for the current year is in the range of $1 million to $1.5 million, with a revenue goal of $2.5 million to be reached in 2 years. The performance goal for the company is to maintain its position as the market leader as measured by gross revenues and customer loyalty (repeat purchases). The company will try to enter its new markets through a series of educational workshops and trade displays at regional and national meetings, along with the release of an educational exercise video.

Market Segmentation Procedures

Market segmentation for this company will include target markets, customer needs, and product-customer fit.

Target Markets

Ideally, SPRI would like to introduce rubber resistance exercise to everyone who is capable of exercising. Aerobics and physical therapy will remain its primary markets, but the new ones will be hospital-based programs, corporate fitness programs, school systems, and senior citizens.

The typical selection criteria that would be applied to determining and identifying target markets do not apply here. Usually, a company must consider demographic and psychographic characteristics, available income, consumer influences, and many other factors that impinge on a consumer's buying decision. The feeling at SPRI is that its products are so unique, affordable, and usable in almost any situation that sophisticated market segmentation procedures are not necessary.

Customer Needs

The bands and the tubing fulfill a definite customer need. Many people do not have access to strength-training equipment, do not want to use that type of equipment, or simply do not have the time to engage in this type of program. The bands and the tubing overcome all these objections because they are inexpensive, portable, safe, and easy to use. These factors, plus an un-conditional, 30-day money-back or replacement guarantee, increase customer loyalty to the products. And, when the products lose their resistance, people reorder them.

Product-Customer Fit

The unlimited potential for the bands would seem to make it difficult to de-velop a good product-customer fit each time, but this is not the case. The bands come in a variety of widths, each having its own tension ratio. The same is true for the tubing as each is color coded to identify its degree of resistance. Every person can therefore select the appropriate product for his or her fitness level. Also, the company knows of no one, including recover-ing cardiac patients, who could not use the bands or tubing to some degree.

Market Analysis

You will note the market analysis for SPRI differs from the health club's only in an assessment of product life cycle as opposed to the industry life cycle analysis completed by the health club.

Market Research

As mentioned previously, SPRI did not conduct a formal market research study last year and will not conduct one this year. This may seem contrary to good marketing practices, but this is not the case for SPRI. The company is con-stantly engaged in informal market research mainly through the written sur-veys and product evaluations that customers complete when they reorder a product. Another method of informal market research is to conduct personal surveys and evaluations at professional trade shows. The results of this research replicate the previous results; that is, everyone is pleased with the products and are willing to refer them to their friends and associates.

Market Demand

The growing demand for SPRI's products is indicated by the doubling of sales revenues every year for the past 3 years. This phenomenal growth rate is ex-pected to continue through the current year. The company sold over $1 mil-lion worth of products last year, and it projects the current year's revenues to be about $1.5 million. This projection reflects the finite life span of the products (and users always reorder) and that new markets are constantly be-ing entered.

It is expected that the market demand for the bands and tubing will continue to grow into the next decade. There is still sufficient growth potential in the existing markets and certainly within the new ones, especially as data from a survey conducted by the International Dance Exercise Association indicated that only 4% of aerobic exercisers had ever used or heard of rubber resistance products.

Product Life Cycle

The product life cycle for the bands and tubing is slightly different from that of the rest of the fitness equipment industry, which is in the growth stage. The bands and tubing are still in the introductory phase. Although many people in the fitness industry are familiar with the products, there are many more who have never heard of rubber resistance equipment. One of SPRI's major marketing efforts will be to educate consumers on the existence of and uses for its products.

Company Analysis

A group of entrepreneurs and physical therapists who felt that an alternative was needed to traditional rehabilitative methods formed SPRI 4 years ago. They wanted this new rehabilitative mechanism to be usable by people at home, in the office, or while traveling. The concept of rubber resistance equipment was made into a reality to provide this alternative method.

The management of SPRI considers itself to be the market leader with a market share between 10% and 15% even though more than 95% of the potential service market is still untapped. The company plans to maintain its leadership position and begin penetrating deeper into the service market by continuing to do simple things well. The company will provide customer services that differentiate it from its competitors. For example, SPRI will ship an order within 24 to 48 hours of receiving it. They also offer a 30-day replacement guarantee on all products, often without asking that the product be returned. (This practice will change in the current year. The company, while continuing to replace worn or broken equipment with no questions asked, will request that the broken band or tubing be sent back so they can determine why it broke.) Finally, SPRI offers its own product liability coverage to anyone who purchases and uses the bands or tubing. Many fitness equipment manufacturers have product liability but do not extend it to the end user.

The geographic service area of SPRI continues to expand. The products are now sold in Japan, Europe, Asia, and Australia, with the United States being the largest consumer market, and SPRI is considering the development of distributorships in these international markets. It plans to service these international accounts as well as they do their domestic ones.

The company determined it had several major strengths that could always be relied on to help it meet these new market demands. The strengths are its small management team, the quality of the products, its commitment to service and excellence, the extension of its product liability insurance to the end users, the characteristics of the products, and the credibility the company gained through networking. Last year, SPRI also began to seek out highly respected professionals involved in all facets of the fitness industry to establish relationships that will be carried into the current year and beyond. These professionals will be used to strengthen the credibility of the corporate team and to provide training workshops for consumers.

The company's strengths and its involvement in many areas of the fitness industry present exciting possibilities. Its corporate management is planning to convert several weaknesses into strengths, the most prevalent being difficulties in quality control over extremely large production runs and the inconsistencies this can lead to in product performance; a small staff, which requires the company to be highly labor intensive; and what SPRI calls a lack of "sophistication." It feels that, because it is growing so rapidly, it needs to start acting as a big company does. This will require more elaborate computerization, developing sales and distribution networks, and hiring more staff members.

Competitor Analysis

There are only a few competitors to SPRI in the rubber resistance area of the fitness industry. None poses a major threat to SPRI. First, these companies are unable to match SPRI's low prices. Also, all these companies and their products were late entrants into the market. A late entrant usually can capitalize on the mistakes of the first provider or can avoid the problems an earlier entrant faced. This was not the case, however, as SPRI has always made such a quality exercise band that none of its competitors tried to copy it. The competitor products have neither the tensile strength, the product liability insurance, nor the replacement guarantee that the SPRI equipment has.

Product Analysis

The company supplies rubber exercise bands in widths ranging from 1/8 to 1 inch. Each width has a different tension that requires a different level of strength to use. The tubing comes in either 4- or 5-foot lengths. The variable tension is identified by color coding. Blue tubing requires the most strength, red and green somewhat less, and yellow the least. Rubber handles make holding on to the tubing easier. The bands are used for upper- and lower-body exercises and the tubing mainly for the upper body.

Marketing Strategies and Tactics

You will note the marketing strategies and tactics portion of this plan follows the format of the health club plan, nearly to the letter. Each company must examine and assess the same market parameters.

Marketing Objectives

The marketing objectives for SPRI for the current year are simple and straightforward. They are:

- to maintain its position as the market leader and its competitive advantage in this niche of the fitness equipment industry by continuing to provide the best possible product at the best possible price with the best customer service of any company in the industry;
- to increase its market share from between 10% and 15% to 20% and to achieve a 25% market share in 2 years;
- to enhance the company's recognition among potential customers in already established markets such as aerobics and rehabilitation;
- to expand the company's reach into new markets, including corporate fitness programs and the medical and chiropractic communities.
- to increase its credibility by creating an advisory network of respected professionals in the fitness industry; and
- to maintain its competitive advantage by appearing at trade shows, offering educational training programs on how to use the bands and tubing properly, and continuing to honor its product warranties and guarantees.

Business Goals

Although SPRI has set no specific dates for completing each business goal, it wants to achieve its goals successfully in the current year. Financially, SPRI is planning to generate revenues of at least $1 million to $1.5 million, with a profit margin of at least 20%. The company will then have a year-end net profit of $200,000 on $1 million in sales. The company wants to continue increasing the size of its sales staff, upgrading from a staff of two salespeople to one of four or five. It wants to improve its distribution methods, perhaps by using overnight air instead of only the United Parcel Service (UPS). Other business goals are to keep personnel expenses under 30% of total expenses and operational expenses under 60% of revenue.

Marketing Strategies

SPRI has devised marketing strategies aimed mainly at the corporate level. The company wants to stay highly visible in the aerobics industry and to increase its visibility in the areas of corporate and hospital-based fitness. It plans to do this by attending, and exhibiting at, trade shows and professional meetings and by providing potential users with complimentary products. The company also spent the latter part of last year searching for contacts in the new markets it wants to penetrate. The strategy for the current year is to meet with these people directly to introduce them to the products.

Other strategies include developing an educational training program for users of the products. Many fitness instructors are currently using the bands and tubing in their exercise classes, and others are using them in their own training workshops for their staff. But not everyone is using the products correctly or in as many ways as they can be used. SPRI plans to provide a series of training workshops and to produce an exercise video in the current year to educate aerobics instructors and corporate fitness leaders on the proper use of the bands and tubing. The company also plans to continue one of its most successful marketing strategies, that is, placing information brochures and flyers in every order they ship. This direct-mail approach has been profitable for the company by generating much product interest and inquiries and has also resulted in repeat and new sales. This is good for the company, but SPRI has neglected to track accurately from which areas most of the inquiries or orders have come. One goal for the current year is to maintain better records of geographic locations for inquires and orders so that other direct-mail campaigns can be more cost-effective.

These corporate strategies lead to two major business strategies for SPRI. Its revenue goal for the current year is between $1 million and $1.5 million. The first way to accomplish this goal is to continue providing superior service to existing accounts. The second way is to attract more major corporate accounts. The difference between a regular account and a major corporate account for SPRI is that a regular account may order anywhere from several to a few hundred bands. A major corporate account, on the other hand, will order 50,000, 100,0000, or even 500,000 bands at a time. SPRI responds to such orders by shipping directly from their manufacturer and by providing the buyer with an even greater discount off the already low price.

The low price of the product has resulted in wide buyer acceptance and approval of the bands and tubing. One thinks that SPRI should consider raising its prices, especially as it is the market leader and since the product life cycle is still in the introductory phase. Fortunately for the consumer, SPRI will not be raising its prices. In fact, the company is constantly working on means to lower the prices even more to make the products available to more end users. Some of SPRI's life-cycle strategies include maintaining its current limited product line and eliminating product imperfections so that when the company enters the growth stage it can concentrate on adding new products, creating new buyers, improving its distribution channels, and developing new promotions and more stable, high-volume discounts. These strategies will help the company to maintain its competitive advantage and to continue as the market leader.

Marketing Tactics

Most of the marketing strategies will be implemented by having company personnel continue their direct-sales approaches, providing quality customer service, and enhancing corporate name recognition by being visible at trade shows and conventions.

Marketing Mix

The marketing mix for SPRI is basic. The products are exercise bands and tubing that are used for conditioning purposes. These products are distributed primarily through the mail as orders are received. There are some retail distribution outlets, but these are under a private label for another company that SPRI will not compete with. SPRI promotes its products at trade shows and national industry conventions, and it distributes complimentary bands and tubing to first-time users at these meetings. SPRI continues to receive much publicity from writers who publish stories about the bands in various publications.

These components of the marketing mix remain virtually stable for SPRI. The only component that can vary is price, and this is usually based on the size of the order. The company offers a step-discount approach to its customers, with larger discounts being offered as the size of the order increases. Bulk orders receive the greatest discounts and are shipped directly from the manufacturer (but the cost accounting goes through SPRI). The company publishes a price list, which it mails with every shipment. There are no hidden costs or upcharges, which is another reason customers remain so loyal. Customers know what the product will cost based on the quantities of their purchases. There are no surprises when they receive the invoice and the products.

Promotional Mix

SPRI, like the Health and Fitness Facility, limits its advertising portion of the promotional mix. However, because it sells a product, not facilities and services limited to a specific area, it must make greater use of advertising. The company uses two types of print ads: full page four color, and 1/3-page black and white. A determination will always be made as to which ads will be placed in a particular trade journal or popular magazine. The company operates with a limited advertising budget, which restricts the number of placements.

Advertising

There will be full-page four-color ads in each I.D.E.A. (International Dance Exercise Association) preconference issue of *Dance Exercise* magazine, which means publication in April/May and September/October. Placements will be made in *American Fitness* to coincide with the AFAA (Aerobics and Fitness Association of America) national show in February, and other smaller placements will be made in each magazine three or four times throughout the remainder of the year. The issues in which these placements will be made has yet to be determined as SPRI is still waiting for readership data from the publisher.

There is one other advertising medium that SPRI will use in the current year. Many catalog houses have requested that the bands be displayed in their mail-order brochures. Orders will come through the catalog houses and monies forwarded to SPRI, which would then distribute the products. This free advertising is invaluable for the company because it will reach an audience they otherwise never could have contacted.

Publicity

Publicity for SPRI's exercise bands and tubing has been phenomenal. National magazines publish articles about the bands or write about exercise programs that use rubber resistance. Aerobics instructors are teaching workshops and including the bands and tubing in their training sessions. Other instructors are making exercise videos and using the bands in their calisthenics segment. There have also been two books published specifically on how to use the bands.

Another group that was introduced to the products late last year was corporate fitness directors. SPRI sponsored a training workshop at a national conference of these directors under the title "Pumping Rubber." The premise of the workshop was to introduce corporate fitness leaders to rubber resistance equipment as an alternative method of strength training for themselves and their employees. SPRI will continue to offer this type of workshop throughout the year, and will negotiate with publishers about producing a book on "pumping rubber."

Public Relations

The public relations efforts of SPRI are simple. The company continues to offer its customers quality products at a low price and to follow up with quality service. The staff is friendly and courteous at all times. The company also enhances its professional public image by displaying at professional trade shows and cosponsoring professional meetings.

Direct Sales

Direct sales is the mainstay of SPRI Products. The company uses direct sales in two ways. First, it exhibits its products at trade shows. The company is willing to give bands away as promotional pieces, but it also is capable of generating a sale during the exhibit. SPRI will now have people who visit their booth fill out information cards or response coupons. This will help determine who visited their booth, where these people came from, whether and how much they purchased, or simply the nature of their inquiries. It also helps with the company's direct-mail campaign, which is its second method of direct sales.

SPRI has a client list of about 2,000 aerobics studios and fitness centers that are considered active clients as they purchase products on a regular basis, or several times a year. When SPRI fills each order, it sends another order form to the client as well as information on new product developments, training workshops, exercise videos, or anything the company may be able to offer. Then a company representative follows up the shipment with a telephone call several days later to see whether the shipment arrived and whether the company can do anything else to assist the customer. This is the most cost-effective way to market the company and its products. SPRI's position as market leader is definitely due to its direct-mail sales, which will continue to be the primary method for marketing and selling the company's products.

Sales Promotions

SPRI does not engage in many standard sales promotions, mainly because the products are already affordably priced. The only type of promotion the company offers is to give free bands to visitors at trade-show exhibits and to attendees at workshops. The reasoning behind this is rather simple. The bands cost SPRI a minimal amount from the manufacturer, and there is always a good possibility of receiving an order from a new client to whom they have provided a free band. SPRI makes the assumption that, even if the person who received the free band does not use it, they still may pass it along to a friend who will possibly order in quantities. The free give-away promotion has been so successful the company rarely uses any other type.

Promotional Mix Summary

The promotional mix for SPRI is based on percentage of effort rather than revenues because most of its marketing budget is allocated to trade shows and exhibits. Thus the breakdown becomes 10% for advertising, 10% for publicity, 15% for public relations, 50% for direct sales, and 15% for sales promotions. These percentages are the predicted, or desired, effort expenditures the company wants to make. However, the figures are flexible and can be modified as the need arises.

Marketing Results

The desired results of the marketing efforts for SPRI for the current year are to achieve $1.5 million in sales revenues with a net profit of approximately 20%, or from $200,000 to $300,000. The company will achieve these results by maintaining its competitive and differential advantages. The competitive advantage will be maintained by continuing to be the price leader in the industry and by providing the best follow-up service. Further activities, such as appearing at trade shows and sponsoring educational workshops, will also help the company keep its competitive advantage.

The differential advantage refers to those qualities of the company that set it apart from its competitors. SPRI differentiates itself by offering bands and tubing in a variety of widths and tensions as well as several auxiliary pieces that allow the user to attach the equipment to chairs and doors. The company will also offer consumers product extensions in the current year, including travel kits that allow the bands and tubing to lie flat in a suitcase or gym bag and different colored bands that provide variable tension even though they are the same width.

The recommendations for the future are that SPRI continues to become more involved in the corporate fitness market, begins to enter into the hospital health and fitness market, and makes an effort to penetrate the markets comprising cardiac rehabilitation and other at-risk populations. The primary recommendation for SPRI's advertising campaign is to decide on a spokesperson for the company, to develop all product literature and ads picturing that spokesperson, and to place the print ads judiciously in the appropriate trade journals.

Chapter 6

The Personal Approach to Sales _

The personal sales approach is usually developed by the company owner or program director to reflect the marketing style, personality, and philosophy of the organization. It will be modified occasionally by sales representatives to fit their individual personalities and various sales situations. These representatives will use the sales approach to sell products, services, and facilities within the appropriate target markets. Because so many avenues of expression are synthesized in the personal sales approach, this final chapter focuses on the personal sales process and its application.

Sales are obviously very important to the future of every company because without sales, revenues cannot be generated. There are two types of sales: the *simple sale* and the *complex sale* (Miller & Heiman, 1985). The simple sale involves a provider selling a program or service to a client once and every repurchase of that service being viewed as another simple sale. For example, you sell health risk appraisals to corporations. Your client decides to test only one department of a corporation at a time. Each time you go back to that client to test another department is a simple sale because the client can discontinue the service at any time.

The complex sale requires that several people, such as the chief executive officer, the personnel director, the benefits manager, and possibly the director of training, give their approval of the purchase before the sale can occur (Miller & Heiman, 1985). This often is the case whenever a health and fitness provider attempts to sell a package of health promotion programs (e.g., stress management, weight control, and smoking cessation) to corporations and/or hospitals.

The Six Steps to a Sale

A good sales program will follow a process, or a series of steps, that results in an exchange between the buyer and the seller. The important thing for every representative of a health and fitness company to learn is that the most effective sales method will use a personal sales approach at the completion of the *sales process*. In personal sales, you, the provider, help the purchaser progress through a series of logical decision-making steps to buy what you are selling. Some of these steps include questions about the need for the program or service, the benefit(s) to be derived from purchasing it, whether the purchase is affordable, how it will be paid for, and whether the purchase will truly satisfy a need. It is the salesperson's responsibility to help the client obtain the answers to these and other questions that may arise, and this is best accomplished by completing the typical sales process (Reibstein, 1985; Sol, 1987).

The best way to increase the probability of a successful personal sales call is to complete the sales process for each prospective client. The sales process has six main steps: *prospecting*, the *approach*, sales *presentation*, handling objections, the *close*, and the follow-up.

Prospecting

Prospecting is the activity whereby the salesperson creates a list of potential customers, or leads, who may be interested in purchasing health and fitness services. Leads can first come from cold contacts with people. Although this method is nonselective and time consuming, it may reveal potential buyers (Reibstein, 1985). Other leads are gained through referrals, responses to advertisements, purchased mailing lists, social and professional contacts, company records, and other salespeople.

A second aspect of prospecting is qualifying the lead. A *qualified lead* is a prospect who has both the willingness and desire to purchase the service and the ability to pay for it. It is unproductive for a salesperson to try to sell programs and services to consumers who cannot afford to purchase them or who have no interest in buying them. Thus the goal of prospecting is to identify qualified leads who can be turned into satisfied clients.

The Approach

The second step in the sales process is the approach. This involves making initial contact with a qualified prospect. Some of the more common methods of approach include sending a direct-mail piece to the client followed by a telephone call, making telephone calls, being introduced by a mutual acquaintance, or simply showing up cold at the prospect's place of business and trying to arrange a meeting. The salesperson should first develop an understanding of what the client wants and needs and how the client perceives what you are selling. This will help determine the sales approach to use. Also, Reibstein (1985) suggests that the first few minutes of the initial meeting be considered part of the approach because the salesperson must gain the prospect's attention, listen to what the prospect is saying about needs that your company can satisfy, arouse curiosity about the program or service, and build the foundation of a mutually beneficial conversation.

The Presentation

The third step involves the actual sales presentation. The basic goals of the presentation are to gain the prospect's attention, to identify or create an interest in the programs or services, to provide evidence that the services can satisfy the client's needs, and then to use this information to assist the prospect in taking action, that is, making a purchase.

The standard sales presentation is designed to show the clients how you think the features of your programs can benefit them and satisfy their needs. But Miller and Heiman (1987) emphatically state that this approach results in more lost sales than in completed ones. They suggest using a client-oriented presentation in which the salesperson listens to the client, identifies the needs to be satisfied, and then modifies the presentation accordingly.

This is where personal selling shows its greatest advantage over mass selling, advertising, and promotion. The salesperson can discuss the program's benefits in terms of the prospect and the identified needs rather than in terms of the program's features. Then the client can make the purchase with a feeling of perceived ownership, which leads to feelings of security about the purchase. It increases the probability that the client will repurchase, and it decreases the probability of objections to the sale.

Handling Objections During the Presentation

The sales presentation that results in a sale is obviously the best possible case. But many sales calls meet with objections, and the salesperson must be prepared to handle them. The salesperson must view objections as opportunities to learn more about the client and as a chance to provide more information that will lead to a sale. The key to handling any type of objection is to listen to what the prospect is really saying. The salesperson who can meet objections and handle them skillfully will make more sales than will the salesperson who has difficulty responding to objections.

Closing the Sale

The next step in the sales process is the actual close. This is when the customer agrees to buy the product. The customer will provide the salesperson with verbal and nonverbal "buying signals." When one of these signals occurs, the salesperson should attempt to close the sale. The closing must explain all the final terms of the sale (such as program contents and costs) and specify delivery dates, delivery sites, and payment methods. It should also include signing a contract that specifies the obligations of each party.

The Follow-Up

The follow-up to the close is vital. It consists of providing all the services that were promised in the sale, providing assistance and service after the sale, and analyzing the customer's postpurchase satisfaction. Follow-up activities often will be the major determinant of the customer repurchasing the services. Follow-up service will also enhance the company's image, identify the client's level of satisfaction, increase the probability of referrals for future sales calls, and create a track record that will make those future sales calls easier to close. It is easy for a health and fitness company to talk about the quality of the follow-up service it provides, but it is much more difficult actually to provide that service. Remember that poor follow-up service may cause the current client not to repurchase and future prospects to look for another provider.

An Example of the Sales Process

The entire sales process can be described by an example. Your company wants to sell health risk appraisals to a major corporate employer who has publicly expressed an interest in developing employee health and fitness programs. This is obviously a qualified prospect. Your sales representative must first identify the initial contact person and whether there are others who must be involved in the purchase decision. Your representative telephones the prospect and asks for the name of the person to whom information about employee health risk appraisals should be sent. Then a letter is written to that person, and, within a week, a telephone call is made to schedule an appointment to discuss the program in person.

Your salesperson arrives at the appointed time dressed professionally and appearing confident. Discussions with the first buyer follow, the conversation is mutually beneficial, all objections are handled properly and to the client's satisfaction, and your representative leaves with a request for a proposal that can be submitted to the other executive decision makers. The proposal should be written and returned to the first buyer, who will forward it to other decision makers and then contact you to schedule meetings with them. The sales presentation will need to be repeated as many times as there are individual meetings, so your salesperson should try to meet the final decision maker as soon as possible. Remember that, before you have closed the sale, the client may have entertained bids by other providers. Therefore, your representative must specify the uniqueness of your program, how it will best satisfy the buyer's particular needs, and then, to close the sale, offer the program at a price that is competitive yet fair. Now it is up to you to provide the program and follow it up with quality service to ensure that the client is satisfied and may purchase other programs and services.

Quality programs that are offered in a client-centered manner (the clients feel they are getting value and service for their money) will give your company an excellent reputation, a significant number of referrals, and a large number of subsequent sales. Some of the service provision strategies you may want to use follow:

- Develop programs and services that are innovative and difficult for competitors to imitate.
- Achieve the lowest cost position relative to the competition by using strategic pricing methods.
- Use market segmentation strategies to develop, package, present, and differentiate services (*service differentiation*).
- Hire qualified staff and develop them into a dedicated staff.
- Provide customer-oriented services through *service proliferation* and *value-added enhancements* that are unique to each client.

The goals of the promotional part of the marketing plan are to create name recognition of the company and awareness of its programs and services and to entice clients to purchase those programs and services. Providing quality service will result in contract renewals as well as new customer referrals. These are additional sales that must be closed and serviced. Finally, the entire marketing process must remain constantly active so that your company can be at the forefront with its health and fitness marketing efforts.

Glossary

Advertising—A paid form of nonpersonal communication by an identified sponsor or advertiser with the purpose of informing the consumer about a product, program, or service

Approach—A step in the sales process when the seller tries to make contact with the buyer

Balance sheet—A financial statement that shows the assets, liabilities, and owner's equity at any given date

Break-even analysis—An analysis conducted on fixed costs (those that remain the same over time) and variable costs (those that change) to determine the point at which there is neither a net profit nor a net loss (i.e., costs equal revenues) and used to determine whether a company can break even on a service at a particular price

Budget—A process and a document that detail the financial aspects of a company

Business plan—A formal, written document that describes a company's activities with respect to achieving its goals

Capital—Although commonly referred to as money available in the assets of the company, also the amount representing the owner's equity in the assets of the company

Cash flow—The amount of money being earned or paid out on a monthly, quarterly, or annual basis

Cash-flow statement—A statement that specifies the cash requirements of a company on a monthly, quarterly,or annual basis

Close—A step in the sales process when the buyer agrees to purchase the program or service

Company analysis—A section of the business plan that details the history and performance of the company for which the plan is being written

Competitive analysis—The process of gathering information about competitors to better specify marketing strategies and tactics

Competitive position—The actual position or rank, described either qualitatively or quantitatively, that a company holds in the market

Competitive pricing—A method of pricing goods and services in a manner similar to other companies in the market

Competitor analysis—An investigation into the performance factors related to the success or failure of a competitor's business and how this may affect the market

Competitors—Businesses offering similar programs and services

Complex sale—Any sale requiring several presentations to a client or where there is more than one purchasing decision maker

Consumer—The purchaser or end user of a program or service

Customers—Those individuals or companies who purchase products, programs, and services

Demographics—Quantifiable information on the characteristics of a selected group of consumers

Development costs—The costs associated with the start-up of a program or a business

Differentiation—The process of identifying company and product characteristics that make each provider unique and lead to an advantageous position in the market

Direct mail—A form of advertising and promotion that involves mailing information to prospective clients

Distribution channel—The method by which providers pass their programs and services along to consumers

Executive summary—The first section of the business and marketing plans which concisely describes the contents of the plan

Financial analysis—A section of the business plan that describes the financial requirements of the company and the monetary constraints under which it will operate

Financial planning—The process of preparing budgets and forecasting monetary requirements of a business

Financial ratios—A variety of calculations used to determine the financial success or failure of a company.

Inventory = sales ÷ inventory

Fixed assets turnover = sales ÷ net fixed assets

Total assets turnover = sales ÷ total assets

Profit margin = net profit after taxes (NPAT) ÷ sales, or profit before taxes (PBT)— sales ÷ sales

Return on investment (ROI) = NPAT ÷ total assets

Follow-up—The final stage of the sales process, in which the seller maintains contact with the buyer to ensure satisfaction and to create an atmosphere conducive to future sales

Forecasting—A method of predicting future growth and sales

Goals—Qualitative, usually long-range, statements about what a company wants to achieve

Industry analysis—A section of the business plan that describes the state of the industry

Industry/product life cycle—A 4-phase description of the path that every program or service must follow: introduction, growth, maturity, and decline

Liquidity—Cash that is readily available or that can be easily obtained:

Current ratio = current assets (CA) ÷ current liabilities (CL)

Quick ratio = CA—inventories ÷ CL

Loss leader—A program or service that is offered at a very low price to get people to buy other, more expensive services

Management analysis—A section of the business plan that describes the personnel who will operate the business

Market—That group of consumers with the ability and willingness to make exchanges or purchases for products, programs, and services

Market analysis—The section of the business and marketing plan that describes the market conditions under which the business must operate

Market attractiveness—The degree to which a company can easily enter a market and probably be successful

Market barriers—Those factors that prevent a company from entering into or exiting from a market

Market demand—The consumer needs and requirements for a given product, program, or service

Market-entry strategies—Those plans and decisions that a company will follow to penetrate a market

Market niche—A group of customers with similar characteristics that is serviced by companies that cannot compete in the larger segments of the market

Market positioning—The way a company places its offerings within a given market

Market research—The systematic process of collecting, analyzing, interpreting, and using relevant data for the purpose of making accurate marketing decisions

Market sales and revenue—The revenue generated by selling a given product in a particular market in a given time frame

Market scope—The area in which a company offers its services

Market segmentation—The process of breaking down the total heterogeneous market into smaller, more homogeneous groups with similar characteristics or needs that the company can more easily satisfy

Market share—The percentage of the market a company "owns" in relation to the total market

Marketing—Information and exchange activities conducted by individuals and companies for the purposes of satisfying consumer needs and marketer's goals

Marketing mix—The composition of the four basic components of any marketing program or strategy involving product, price, place, and promotions

Marketing plan—The formal written document that describes all the activities a company will engage in to inform the public about its products and to convince them to buy

Marketing strategies—The process of selecting a target market and the appropriate marketing mix variables that will lead to maximum satisfaction of consumers in that market

Marketing tactics—Those actions that are instituted to make a given marketing strategy successful

Media—The vehicle or medium for conveying a message such as print, television, radio, billboards, and word of mouth

Mission statement—A statement of purpose about what the company plans to do to achieve its goals

Networking—The process of meeting other people who possess skills and contacts that will help conduct a business

Nonprice competition—The development of programs and services with such a high perceived value and quality that actual costs do not enter into the buying decision

Objectives—Performance-based, measurable, short-range statements about what a company wants to achieve within a given time frame

Operational expenses—The money required to conduct the business

Performance indicators—Those factors that help determine whether a company will achieve its goals and objectives

Presentation—A step in the sales process when the information about a service is provided for the client

Price—The value of programs or services agreed on by consumers and providers in the exchange process

Primary data—Information collected to analyze a specific situation, being either qualitative (subjective) or quantitative (measurable)

Pro forma—A projection, most commonly used with reference to financial statements and staffing requirements

Product advertising—The conveying of information about a tangible offering that has need-satisfying capabilities

Profit-and-loss statement—A financial record or document that shows a company's performance (whether it made or lost money) over a specified period of time, usually monthly or annually

Promotion—Activities that inform the buying public of the existence of a program or service and its need-satisfying capabilities and that allow the consumer to try the service at little or no cost

Promotional mix—The combination of advertising, promotions, publicity, public relations, and sales that is used to market programs and services and to convince consumers of their need-satisfying capabilities

Prospecting—The process of identifying possible clients

Provider—The individual or company that offers services

Public relations—An organized communication program with various target groups designed to enhance a company's image and reputation in the community

Publicity—Any nonpersonal communication in the media that stimulates consumer demand and is not paid for by the company

Qualified lead—Those prospective clients who have been identified as most likely to purchase and who have the means to make a purchase

Sales—The process by which the company assists the consumer in a buying decision

Sales process—The 6-step method—prospecting, approach, presentation, handling objections, close, and follow-up—that every company must follow to secure a client

Sales promotions—Marketing activities and communications, such as discounts and incentives, that stimulate consumer interest and purchasing behaviors

Secondary data—Information that has been collected for purposes other than those related to the research project currently undertaken (sources can be internal or external)

Service advertising—The conveying of information about an intangible offering that has need-satisfying capabilities

Service differentiation—The separation of one company's services from its competitors by real, imagined, or perceived characteristics

Service marketing—A unique aspect of marketing in which the product is intangible and results are based on customer perception and satisfaction

Service proliferation—An increase in the type and number of offerings made by a company

Simple sale—A sale in which the decision to buy is made by only one person

Strategic analysis—A section of the business plan that describes the strategies and tactics a company will engage in to achieve its goals and objectives

Strategies—Conceptual plans or methods that will help achieve goals and objectives

SWOT analysis—A part of the company analysis that identifies strengths, weaknesses, opportunities, and threats

Tactics—The methods used to achieve goals and objectives

Target market—The market segment at which a company aims a specific marketing effort or strategy

Telemarketing—The use of telecommunications to inform consumers about programs and services

Value-added enhancements—Characteristics or properties that are added to a program or service to increase its perceived value and possibly its price

Word of mouth—Verbal communication between people about a company or its programs or services

References _____

Ardell, D.B. (1986). *High level wellness* (2nd ed.). Berkeley, CA: Ten Speed Press.

Assael, H. (1985). *Marketing management: Strategy and action.* Belmont, CA: Wadsworth.

Bagozzi, R.P. (1986a). *Principles of marketing management.* Chicago: Science Research Associates.

Bagozzi, R.P. (1986b). Marketing management: Strategies, tactics, new horizons. In G.E. Germane (Ed.), *The executive course: What every manager needs to know about the essentials of business* (pp. 1-66). Reading, MA: Addison-Wesley.

Bellingham, R., & Tager, M.J. (1986). *Designing effective health promotion programs: The 20 skills for success.* Chicago, IL: Great Performance.

Bennett, P.D. (1988). *Marketing.* New York: McGraw-Hill.

Buzzell, R.D., & Gale, B.T. (1987). *The PIMS principles: Linking strategy to performance.* New York: Free Press.

Caro, R.M. (1986). *Financial management.* Boston: International Racquet Sports Association.

Chenoweth, D.H. (1987). *Planning health promotion at the worksite.* Indianapolis: Benchmark Press.

Clair, K.M. (1987, July/August). Operating standards define effectiveness. *Optimal Health,* pp. 52-53, 56, 58.

Cohen, W.A. (1987). *Developing a winning marketing plan.* New York: Wiley.

Crego, E.T., Deaton, B., & Schiffrin, P.D. (1986). *How to write a business plan.* American Management Association.

Gardner, J.R., Rachlin, R., & Sweeny, H.W.A. (Eds.) (1986). *Handbook of strategic planning.* New York: Wiley.

Gerson, R.F. (1987, April). Marketing to corporations: Road MAPS for success. *Club Business,* pp. 53-54.

Hamermesh, R.G. (1986). *Making strategy work.* New York: Wiley.

International Racquet Sports Association. (1985). *Why people join.* Boston: Author.

King, W.C. (1986). Formulating strategies and contingency plans. In J.R. Gardner, R. Rachlin, & H.W.A. Allen (Eds.), *Handbook of strategic planning* (pp. 6.1-6.30). New York: Wiley.

Kizer, W.M. (1987). *The healthy workplace*. New York: Wiley.

Kotler, P. (1988). *Marketing management: Analysis, planning, implementation and control*. Englewood Cliffs, NJ: Prentice-Hall.

Leza, R.L., & Placenia, J.F. (1982). *Develop your business plan*. Sunnyvale, CA: Oasis Press.

Marcus, B.W. (1986). *Competing for clients: The complete guide to marketing and promoting professional services*. Chicago: Probus.

Marrus, S.K. (1984). *Building the strategic plan: Find, analyze and present the right information*. New York: Wiley.

Miller, R.B., & Heiman, S.E. (1985). *Strategic selling*. New York: Morrow.

Miller, R.B., & Heiman, S.E. (1987). *Conceptual selling*. New York: Morrow.

Mulvihill, D.F., & Konopa, L.J. (1986). Developing price policies. In V. Buell (Ed.), *Handbook of modern marketing* (pp. 29.3-29.10). New York: McGraw-Hill.

Murphy, P.E., & Enis, B.M. (1985). *Marketing*. Glenview, IL: Scott Foresman.

O'Donnell, M.P. (1986). Definition of health promotion. *American Journal of Health Promotion*, **1**, 4.

Opatz, J.P. (1985). *A primer of health promotion*. Washington, DC: Oryn.

Opatz, J.P. (Ed.) (1987). *Health promotion evaluation: Measuring the organizational impact*. Stevens Point, WI: National Wellness Institute/ National Wellness Association.

Parkinson, R.S. (1982). *Managing health promotion in the workplace*. Palo Alto, CA: Mayfield.

Patton, R.W., Corry, J.M., Gettman, L.R., & Graf, J.S. (1986). *Implementing health/fitness programs*. Champaign, IL: Human Kinetics Publishers.

Patton, R.W., Grantham, W., Gerson, R.F., & Gettman, L.R. (1989). *Developing and managing health/fitness facilities*. Champaign, IL: Human Kinetics Publishers.

Peters, T.J. (1987). *Thriving on chaos*. New York: Knopf.

Rapp, S., & Collins, T. (1987). *MaxiMarketing*. New York: McGraw-Hill.

Reibstein, D.J. (1985). *Marketing: Concepts, strategies, and decisions*. Englewood Cliffs, NJ: Prentice-Hall.

Ries, A., & Trout, J. (1986). *Positioning: The battle for your mind*. New York: McGraw-Hill.

Rink, D.R., & Swan, J.E. (1987). Fitting business strategic and tactical planning to the product life cycle. In W.R. King & D.I. Cleland (Eds.), *Strategic planning and managing handbook* (pp. 352-373). New York: Van Nostrand Reinhold.

Settle, R.B., & Alreck, P.L. (1986). *Why they buy*. New York: Wiley.

Sol, N. (1987, November/December). Sales sophistication needed for growth. *Optimal Health*, p. 11.

Steiner, G.A. (1979). *Strategic planning*. New York: Free Press.

Strategies for integrating health care. (1987, March/April special issue). *Optimal Health*,

Weinrauch, J.D. (1987). *The marketing problem solver*. New York: Wiley.

Suggested Reading List

Ardell, D.B., & Tager, M.J. (1982). *Planning for wellness*. Dubuque, IA: Kendall/Hunt.

Bellingham, R., & Tager, M.J. (1986). *Designing effective health promotion programs: The 20 skills for success*. Chicago: Great Performance.

Bennett, P.D. (1988). *Marketing*. New York: McGraw-Hill.

Buell, V.P. (1986). *Handbook of modern marketing*. New York: McGraw-Hill.

Chenoweth, D.H. (1987). *Planning health promotion at the worksite*. Indianapolis: Benchmark Press.

Cohen, W.A. (1987). *Developing a winning market plan*. New York: Wiley.

Gardner, J.R., Rachlin, R., & Sweeny, H.W.A. (Eds.) (1986). *Handbook of strategic planning*. New York: Wiley.

Hamermesh, R.G. (1986). *Making strategy work*. New York: Wiley.

King, W.R., & Cleland, D.I. (1987). *Strategic planning and management handbook*. New York: Van Nostrand Reinhold.

Kizer, W.M. (1987). *The healthy workplace*. New York: Wiley.

Kotler, P. (1988). *Marketing Management: Analysis, Planning, Implementation, and Control*. Englewood Cliffs, NJ: Prentice-Hall.

O'Donnell, M.P., & Ainsworth, T. (1984). *Health promotion in the work place*. New York: Wiley.

Opatz, J.P. (1985). *A primer of health promotion*. Washington, DC: Oryn Publications.

Strategies for integrating health care. (1987, March/April special issue). *Optimal Health*.

Parkinson, R.S. (1982). *Managing health promotion in the workplace*. Palo Alto, CA: Mayfield.

Patton, R.W., Grantham, W., Gerson, R.F., & Gettman, L.R. (1989). *Developing and managing health/fitness facilities*. Champaign, IL: Human Kinetics Publishers.

Rapp, S., & Collins, T. (1987). *Maximarketing*. New York: McGraw-Hill.

Settle, R.B., & Alreck, P.L. (1986). *Why they buy*. New York: Wiley.

Index _____

A
Action plan, 26
Activity services, 53
Advertising, 23, 65, 69, 73, 75
  direct mail, 3, 20, 23, 74
  product, 70
  service, 12
  word of mouth, 70
Analysis
  break-even, 36, 42
  company, 7, 8, 10
  competitive, 12, 57
  financial, 9, 25, 36
  industry, 7, 8, 14, 16
  management, 9, 25, 31
  market, 7, 8, 16, 56
  strategic, 8, 25
  SWOT, 9, 10, 59

B
Balance sheet, 36
Budget, 23, 36, 38, 40, 42
Business plan, 1, 4-5, 7 (*see also* Sample business plan)
Buying signals, 106

C
Capital, 36
Cash flow, 6, 36, 38
Communication, 67
Competitive position, 13
Competitive pricing, 22